Diabetes

Editors

KIM ZUBER
JANE S. DAVIS

PHYSICIAN ASSISTANT CLINICS

www.physicianassistant.theclinics.com

Consulting Editor
JAMES A. VAN RHEE

April 2020 • Volume 5 • Number 2

ELSEVIER

1600 John F. Kennedy Boulevard • Suite 1800 • Philadelphia, Pennsylvania, 19103-2899

http://www.theclinics.com

PHYSICIAN ASSISTANT CLINICS Volume 5, Number 2
April 2020 ISSN 2405-7991, ISBN-13: 978-0-323-70918-7

Editor: Katerina Heidhausen
Developmental Editor: Casey Potter

Physician Assistant Clinics (ISSN: 2405–7991) is published quarterly by Elsevier Inc., 360 Park Avenue South, New York, NY 10010-1710. Months of issue are January, April, July, and October. Periodicals postage paid at New York, NY and additional mailing offices. Subscription prices are $150.00 per year (US individuals), $216.00 (US institutions), $100.00 (US students), $150.00 (Canadian individuals), $271.00 (Canadian institutions), $100.00 (Canadian students), $150.00 (international individuals), $271.00 (international institutions), and $100.00 (international students). Foreign air speed delivery is included in all *Clinics* subscription prices. All prices are subject to change without notice. POSTMASTER: Send address changes to *Physician Assistant Clinics*, Elsevier Periodicals Customer Service, 11830 Westline Industrial Drive, St. Louis, MO 63146. Customer Service Health Sciences Division, Subscription Customer Service, 3251 Riverport Lane, Maryland Heights, MO 63043. **Customer Service: 1-800-654-2452 (U.S. and Canada); 314-447-8871 (outside U.S. and Canada). Fax: 314-447-8029. E-mail: journalscustomerservice-usa@elsevier.com (for print support); journalsonlinesupport-usa@elsevier.com (for online support).**

Reprints. For copies of 100 or more, of articles in this publication, please contact the Commercial Reprints Department, Elsevier Inc., 360 Park Avenue South, New York, NY 10010-1710. Tel. 212-633-3874; Fax: 212-633-3820; E-mail: reprints@elsevier.com.

Physician Assistant Clinics is covered in *EMBASE/Excerpta Medica* and *ESCI*.

PROGRAM OBJECTIVE
The goal of the *Physician Assistant Clinics* is to keep practicing physician assistants up to date with current clinical practice by providing timely articles reviewing the state of the art in patient care.

TARGET AUDIENCE
Physician Assistants and other healthcare professionals

LEARNING OBJECTIVES
Upon completion of this activity, participants will be able to:
1. Review the epidemiology, pathophysiology, and clinical manifestations for various Diabetes classification types
2. Discuss recommended best practices and evidence-based care for the treatment and management of the patient with Diabetes
3. Recognize the clinical presentation, complications, diagnostic evaluation and management of Diabetes in select population groups

ACCREDITATION
The Elsevier Office of Continuing Medical Education (EOCME) is accredited by the Accreditation Council for Continuing Medical Education (ACCME) to provide continuing medical education for physicians.

The EOCME designates this journal-based CME activity for a maximum of 15 *AMA PRA Category 1 Credit*(s)™. Physicians should claim only the credit commensurate with the extent of their participation in the activity.

All other healthcare professionals requesting continuing education credit for this enduring material will be issued a certificate of participation.

DISCLOSURE OF CONFLICTS OF INTEREST
The EOCME assesses conflict of interest with its instructors, faculty, planners, and other individuals who are in a position to control the content of CME activities. All relevant conflicts of interest that are identified are thoroughly vetted by EOCME for fair balance, scientific objectivity, and patient care recommendations. EOCME is committed to providing its learners with CME activities that promote improvements or quality in healthcare and not a specific proprietary business or a commercial interest.

The planning committee, staff, authors and editors listed below have identified no financial relationships or relationships to products or devices they or their spouse/life partner have with commercial interest related to the content of this CME activity:
Sumera Ahmed, MD, BC-ADM; Molly E. Band, MHS, PA-C; Esther Bennitta; Courtney Lee Bennett Wilke, MPAS, PA-C; Sarah V. Cogle, PharmD, BCCCP; Jane S. Davis, MSN, DNP; Megan J. Dougan, MPAS, PA-C; Brittany M. Dowdle, BA; Joy A. Dugan, DHSc, MPH, PA-C; Harvey A. Feldman, MD, FACP; Katerina Heidhausen; Amber M. Hutchison, PharmD, BCPS, BCGP; Gerald Kayingo, PhD, MMSc, PA-C; Marilu Kelly, MSN, RN, CNE, CHCP; Sarah Dion Kelly, MS, RD, CDE; Rebecca A. Maxson, PharmD, BCPS; Emily K. McCoy, PharmD, BCACP; Virginia McCoy Hass, RN, DNP, FNP-C, PA-C; Ciara Mitchell, MA, RD; Ashley Klaczak Mudra, MPAS, PA-C; Stephanie L. Neary, MPA, MMS, PA-C; Alicia Ottmann, MMS, PA-C; Rosalyn Perry, MPH(c), PA-S; Casey Potter; Melissa Rodzen, MMS, PA-C; Kristen A. Scheckel, PA-C; James A. Van Rhee, MS, PA-C; Margarita Vincent, MPH(c), PA-S; Heidi M. Webb, MMS, PA-C, AAPA, ASEPA; Clipper F. Young, PharmD, MPH, CDE, BC-ADM, BCGP; Kim Zuber, PA-C, MS

UNAPPROVED/OFF-LABEL USE DISCLOSURE
The EOCME requires CME faculty to disclose to the participants:
1. When products or procedures being discussed are off-label, unlabelled, experimental, and/or investigational (not US Food and Drug Administration [FDA] approved); and
2. Any limitations on the information presented, such as data that are preliminary or that represent ongoing research, interim analyses, and/or unsupported opinions. Faculty may discuss information about pharmaceutical agents that is outside of FDA-approved labelling. This information is intended solely for CME and is not intended to promote off-label use of these medications. If you have any questions, contact the medical affairs department of the manufacturer for the most recent prescribing information.

TO ENROLL

The CME program is available to all *Physician Assistant Clinics* subscribers at no additional fee. To subscribe to the *Physician Assistant Clinics*, call customer service at 1-800-654-2452 or sign up online at www.physicianassistant.theclinics.com.

METHOD OF PARTICIPATION

In order to claim credit, participants must complete the following:

1. Complete enrolment as indicated above
2. Read the activity
3. Complete the CME Test and Evaluation. Participants must achieve a score of 70% on the test. All CME Tests and Evaluations must be completed online

CME INQUIRIES/SPECIAL NEEDS

For all CME inquiries or special needs, please contact elsevierCME@elsevier.com.

Contributors

CONSULTING EDITOR

JAMES A. VAN RHEE, MS, PA-C
Associate Professor, Program Director, Yale School of Medicine, Yale Physician Assistant Online Program, New Haven, Connecticut

EDITORS

KIM ZUBER, PA-C, MS
Executive Director, American Academy of Nephrology PAs, St Petersburg, Florida

JANE S. DAVIS, MSN, DNP
Division of Nephrology, The University of Alabama at Birmingham, Birmingham, Alabama

AUTHORS

SUMERA AHMED, MD, BC-ADM
Assistant Professor and Diabetologist, College of Osteopathic Medicine, Touro University California, Vallejo, California

MOLLY E. BAND, MHS, PA-C
Department of Pediatric Nephrology, Connecticut Children's Medical Center, Hartford, Connecticut

COURTNEY LEE BENNETT WILKE, MPAS, PA-C
Assistant Professor, School of Physician Assistant Practice, College of Medicine, Florida State University, Tallahassee, Florida

SARAH V. COGLE, PharmD, BCCCP
Pharmacy Practice Department, Assistant Clinical Professor, Auburn University Harrison School of Pharmacy, Auburn, Alabama

MEGAN J. DOUGAN, MPAS, PA-C
Fairview, Pennsylvania

BRITTANY M. DOWDLE, BA
Suches, Georgia

JOY A. DUGAN, DHSc, MPH, PA-C
Associate Program Director, Joint MSPAS/MPH Program, Touro University California, Vallejo, California

HARVEY A. FELDMAN, MD, FACP
Professor, Physician Assistant Program, Nova Southeastern University, Fort Lauderdale, Florida

AMBER M. HUTCHISON, PharmD, BCPS, BCGP
Pharmacy Practice Department, Associate Clinical Professor, Auburn University Harrison School of Pharmacy, Auburn, Alabama

GERALD KAYINGO, PhD, MMSc, PA-C
Health Sciences Associate Clinical Professor, Betty Irene Moore School of Nursing, University of California, Davis, Sacramento, California

SARAH DION KELLY, MS, RD, CDE
Inova Center for Wellness and Metabolic Health, Fairfax, Virginia

REBECCA A. MAXSON, PharmD, BCPS
Assistant Clinical Professor, Auburn University Harrison School of Pharmacy, Auburn, Alabama

EMILY K. McCOY, PharmD, BCACP
Associate Clinical Professor, Auburn University Harrison School of Pharmacy, Mobile, Alabama

VIRGINIA McCOY HASS, RN, DNP, FNP-C, PA-C
Health Sciences Associate Clinical Professor, Betty Irene Moore School of Nursing, University of California, Davis, Sacramento, California

CIARA MITCHELL, MA, RD
Adjunct Instructor, Department of Human Studies, The University of Alabama at Birmingham, Birmingham, Alabama

ASHLEY KLACZAK MUDRA, MPAS, PA-C
Physician Assistant, North Florida Integrative Medicine, Gainesville, Florida

STEPHANIE L. NEARY, MPA, MMS, PA-C
Instructor and Didactic Coordinator, Physician Assistant Online Program, Yale University, New Haven, Connecticut

ALICIA OTTMANN, MMS, PA-C
Clinician Services Manager, Neighborhood Outreach Access to Health - HonorHealth, Phoenix, Arizona

ROSALYN PERRY, MPH(c), PA-S
Student, Joint MSPAS/MPH Program, Touro University California, Vallejo, California

MELISSA RODZEN, MMS, PA-C
American Academy of Physician Assistants, Alexandria, Virginia; American Association of Clinical Endocrinologists, Jacksonville, Florida; American Diabetes Association, Arlington, Virginia

KRISTEN A. SCHECKEL, PA-C
Creekside Endocrine Associates, Denver, Colorado

MARGARITA VINCENT, MPH(c), PA-S
Student, Joint MSPAS/MPH Program, Touro University California, Vallejo, California

HEIDI M. WEBB, MMS, PA-C, AAPA, ASEPA
Senior Physician Assistant, Endocrinology and Internal Medicine, Bahl and Bahl Medical Associates, Pittsburgh, Pennsylvania

CLIPPER F. YOUNG, PharmD, MPH, CDE, BC-ADM, BCGP
Assistant Professor, Clinical Pharmacist, College of Osteopathic Medicine, Touro University California, Vallejo, California

Contents

As the number of patients with diabetes is rising nationwide along, with concurrent advancement of screening and diagnostic testing, the medical community is now able to understand diabetes beyond type 1 diabetes mellitus and type 2 diabetes mellitus. This guide reviews the laboratory testing available and the diagnostic criteria for many classifications of diabetes. Hemoglobin A1c has long been considered the ideal screening tool for diabetes, but it is not always accurate. When hemoglobin A1c is not reliable, other screening tests must be used. Practitioners should be familiar with the available testing and the clinical indications for the utilization of these diagnostics.

The pathophysiology of type 2 diabetes mellitus is characterized by interrelated deficits observed in the liver, muscle, brain, adipose tissue, kidneys, gastrointestinal tract, and pancreas. Insulin resistance and β cell dysfunction progress along a spectrum of disease from hyperinsulinemia to impaired glucose tolerance, hyperglycemia, and frank insulin deficiency. Understanding the relationships between these multiple shortcomings will help clinicians target treatment using different approaches that are effective for each patient's unique presentation. Early and intensive interventions improve outcomes and limit long-term complications.

Diabetes is a complex, multifactorial disease that permeates every aspect of a patient's life and often the lives of their friends and families. While managing a disease that heavily depends on lifestyle choices, a patient-centered care model is essential. Providers should use a variety of strategies focused on patient-specific goals and barriers while developing a detailed, individualized care plan.

devastating consequences, and because of their emergent nature, require prompt recognition and competent management. These complications are diabetic ketoacidosis, hyperosmolar hyperglycemic state, also known as hyperosmolar hyperglycemic nonketotic state, and hypoglycemia. They represent extremes in the spectrum of dysglycemia. This review provides current clinically relevant information on the epidemiology, pathogenesis, causes, clinical presentation, and management of these conditions.

The day-to-day life of a patient with diabetes can be daunting. Over the years, chronic complications arise and involving almost all systems of the body. Common chronic complications of diabetes include atherosclerotic diseases, retinopathy, neuropathy, and nephropathy. Additionally, patients with diabetes are at increased risk for oral health problems, skin conditions, susceptibility to infections, genitourinary complications, and comorbid depression. This article focuses on the recognition, management, and prevention of these chronic complications of diabetes. We also discuss the importance of glycemic control and routine health maintenance. We recommend a patient-centered team-based approach to improve outcomes.

Gestational diabetes mellitus (GDM): glucose intolerance with first onset or recognition during pregnancy. GDM is diagnosed with increased frequency, and maternal hyperglycemia has a direct connection to adverse pregnancy outcomes. GDM places increased burden on the mother and fetus not only in the peri-partum state, but long term. Recent findings support earlier screening and use of biomarkers in diagnosing GDM. Gold standard of treatment remains lifestyle modifications of nutrition therapy, physical activity, and self-monitoring blood glucose. Insulin therapy remains the gold standard in patients requiring pharmacotherapy. Women with GDM need long-term follow-up with continued lifestyle modification and risk mitigation.

Diabetes mellitus is a complex group of metabolic disorders characterized by a chronically elevated blood glucose level, which can result from either a defect in insulin secretion, a defect in insulin responsiveness, or both. Although there are many similarities between diabetes in adults and diabetes in children, there are significant differences in diagnosis, presentation, and treatment in the pediatric population. This article focuses on pediatric-specific aspects of diabetes.

PHYSICIAN ASSISTANT CLINICS

SERIES OF RELATED INTEREST

Endocrinology and Metabolism Clinics of North America
https://www.endo.theclinics.com/
Medical Clinics of North America
https://www.medical.theclinics.com/
Primary Care: Clinics in Office Practice
https://www.primarycare.theclinics.com/

THE CLINICS ARE AVAILABLE ONLINE!
Access your subscription at:
www.theclinics.com

Foreword

Diabetes: By the Numbers

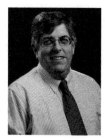

James A. Van Rhee, MS, PA-C
Consulting Editor

According to the Centers for Disease Control and Prevention National Diabetes Statistics Report: 2017,[1] there are 30.3 million US adults with diabetes, and 1 in 4 do not know they have diabetes. In the United States, 84.1 million adults have prediabetes, that is 1 in 3 have prediabetes, and 90% do not know they have prediabetes. Prediabetes is noted in 23.1 million adults over age 65.

Diabetes is the seventh leading cause of death in the United States. Diabetes is the number one cause of kidney failure, lower-limb amputations, and adult blindness. Finally, in the last 20 years, the number of adults diagnosed with diabetes has more than doubled.

The health care cost burden, total direct and indirect estimated cost, of diagnosed diabetes in the United States in 2012 was $245 billion.[2] The average cost for medical care for a diabetic patient, attributed to their diabetes, is $7900 per year.[2] After adjusting for age and sex, the average medical expenditures for people with diagnosed diabetes are about 2.3 times higher than expenditures for people without diabetes.[2]

This issue of *Physician Assistant Clinics* offers the health care provider the information needed to better care for the diabetic patient and in the long run have a positive effect on the numbers noted above. Zuber and Davis, and a team of experts, provide several excellent articles. Articles in this issue cover the treatment of diabetes, managing chronic complications, and the care of the diabetic patient across the lifespan. For the historical buff, there is an article on diabetes in the twenty-first century and the centennial history of insulin.

Physician Assist Clin 5 (2020) xiii–xiv
https://doi.org/10.1016/j.cpha.2020.01.002
2405-7991/20/© 2020 Published by Elsevier Inc.

I hope you enjoy this issue. Our next issue will cover Hospice and Palliative Care Medicine.

James A. Van Rhee, MS, PA-C
Yale School of Medicine
Yale Physician Assistant Online Program
100 Church Street South, Suite A230
New Haven, CT 06519, USA

E-mail address:
james.vanrhee@yale.edu

Website:
http://www.paonline.yale.edu

REFERENCES

1. Centers for Disease Control and Prevention. National diabetes statistics report, 2017. Atlanta (GA): Centers for Disease Control and Prevention, US Department of Health and Human Services; 2017.
2. American Diabetes Association. Economic costs of diabetes in the US in 2012. Diabetes Care 2013;36(4):1033–46.

A Century of Discovery
The Centennial of Insulin

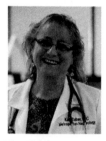 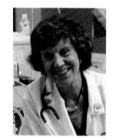

Kim Zuber, PA-C, MS   Jane S. Davis, MSN, DNP
Editors

HAPPY BIRTHDAY INSULIN!

Imagine watching a loved one waste away. This, despite a voracious appetite, unquenchable thirst, and seemingly endless urination. This is a picture of a patient with diabetes prior to the early 1900s.

Although diabetes was described as early as 552 BCE, there was little to do but watch the person with diabetes become more and more debilitated, finally slipping into a coma and death.

In 1869, Dr Paul Langerhans discovered insulin-producing cells in the pancreas but was unable to identify a mechanism to isolate and deliver the product to patients. It was named *inulin*, after the islets.[1]

In 1920, Dr Frederick Banting, a fledgling Toronto orthopedic surgeon whose new practice was not developing, had plenty of time on his hands. He took the opportunity to use laboratory space and 10 dogs to try and discover how to isolate inulin (renamed *insulin* in later years), deliver it, and ameliorate the effects of diabetes.[2] A young chemist, Charles Best, assisted.

Through a series of trial and error attempts, and an unknown number of dogs, they finally succeeded in 1921 with a dog named Marjorie. After Marjorie had her pancreas removed and developed diabetes, she was successfully treated with a substrate of her pancreas and lived 70 days.[2]

From 1920 to 1922, Best and Banting attempted to isolate and purify their serum for the jump from dogs to humans. They attempted to give it as a liquid, as a solid, orally, rectally, intramuscularly, subcutaneously, and by inhalation. Only the injectable mode seemed to work, although, due to purification issues, there were several abscesses along the way and multiple dogs did not survive. After believing they had a clean serum, they made the jump to humans in January 1922. A 14-year-old boy, Leonard Thompson, was the first patient. His recovery astounded his doctors and, in no time, the wonder drug was being used and hailed as a miracle.[2] Imagine a hospital ward with 60 dying children in various stages of diabetic coma. The children's grieving

Physician Assist Clin 5 (2020) xv–xvii
https://doi.org/10.1016/j.cpha.2019.11.001

families surround the bedsides helpless to do anything but watch their children die. Enter a group of men who inject each child with the new wonder drug. Before they reach the last child, the first children injected were waking up to the joy and excitement of their families.

Stories abound from the introduction of insulin. Shortages occurred and there was a need for a purification process. Banting believed no one should make money off insulin and sold the rights for production to the University of Toronto for $1.

There were issues with batch to batch potency. One of Banting's classmates, Dr Joseph Gilchrist was an early user of insulin but dosing was haphazard due to the potency issues. Dr Gilchrist's patients had to go to the local constabulary to bail out the good doctor after an episode of hypoglycemia caused him to be arrested for drunk and disorderly conduct. Although this may have been the first time a hypoglycemic patient was misidentified as drunk, it would not be the last!

Over the next couple years, insulin was refined and standardized, long-acting forms were developed in the 1930s and recombinant DNA human insulin was developed in 1978. The discovery of insulin won the Nobel Prize in Physiology or Medicine in 1923.

Foreshadowing things to come, in a 1929 account of the discovery of insulin, Dr Banting observed, "overfeeding with the lack of exercise predisposes patients to diabetes."[3]

Now, we come full circle. It has been 100 years since the discovery of insulin and to celebrate, we have put together an issue specializing in diabetes with physician assistant, medical doctor, pharmacy, and dietary experts. Neary and Ottman start off with a discussion of how to diagnose diabetes in the twenty-first century. Once diagnosed, the pathophysiology of the disease needs to be understood, and Kelly and Neary walk us through it. In this era of patient-centered care, Rodzen highlights how to make sure the whole patient is treated, not just the disease. Mitchell explains the diet, with highlights on how to adjust to both patient preference and food availability. Pharmacists are invaluable to managing a patient with diabetes, and Maxson and McCoy discuss the oral diabetic medications while Cogle and Hutchison explain all the injectable medications now available. If Banting could see the variety available 100 years after his discovery, his head would spin.

Dugan, Ahmed, Vincent, Perry, and Young show the incredible variations of electronic and digital applications for patients and practitioners. Feldman, Kayingo, and Hass discuss the all too common complications that can occur in a patient with diabetes, both chronic and acute. Never forgetting that patients have lives too, Webb reviews the pregnant patient with diabetes while Band discusses a whole different kettle of fish, the child with diabetes. As the population ages and diabetes occurs more frequently in the older population, Mudra discusses the specific needs of the elderly or infirm. There cannot be a review without looking at the cost of diabetes from both personal and societal points of view by Scheckel. This issue ends with a fun article: Wilke, Dowdle, and Dougan look to the future and predict what the next 100 years will bring. What a shame we will not see how accurate they are in their prognostications!

On this 100th anniversary, the authors thank all the patients who have volunteered as trial subjects, teaching models, and training for generations of practitioners over the past 100 years. The huge leaps in knowledge are due only to the patients encountered over the years. They have also taught us that far from being a diabetic patients, they instead are patients who have diabetes, with patient and not disease state first and foremost. We want to thank all the authors for their expertise and the knowledge that they are sharing. We hope that readers enjoy reading this issue as much as we have enjoyed putting it together.

Happy 100th birthday insulin.

ACKNOWLEDGMENTS

The authors wish to thank C.J. Chun, PAC, MS, without whom this issue would not be possible. C.J.: you are our guiding light.

DISCLOSURE

The authors have no relationships to disclose.

Kim Zuber, PA-C, MS
American Academy of Nephrology PAs
St Petersburg, FL 33707, USA

Jane S. Davis, MSN, DNP
Division of Nephrology
University of Alabama at Birmingham
Birmingham, AL 35223, USA

E-mail addresses:
zuberkim@yahoo.com (K. Zuber)
jsdavis@uabmc.edu (J.S. Davis)

REFERENCES

1. Quianzon CC, Cheikh IE. History of current non-insulin medications for diabetes mellitus. J Community Hosp Intern Med Perspect 2012;2(3).
2. Bliss M. The discovery of insulin 25th anniversary edition. Chicago: University of Chicago Press; 1982.
3. Banting F. The history of insulin. Edinburg Med Journal 1929;36(1):1–18.

Diagnostic Approach to Differentiating Diabetes Types

Stephanie L. Neary, MPA, MMS, PA-C[a],*, Alicia Ottmann, MMS, PA-C[b]

KEYWORDS

- Diabetes mellitus • Diabetes diagnostics • Hemoglobin A_{1c} • Fasting blood glucose
- Monogenic diabetes

KEY POINTS

- Diabetes is a complex disease with many classifications that help differentiate the underlying etiology of hyperglycemia. Understanding the different laboratory tests available and utilizing these as part of a comprehensive evaluation are essential to reaching a correct diagnosis.
- There are many situations and comorbidities that have an impact on laboratory test levels, but in each of these situations, there are additional tests available to aid in the diagnosis of diabetes.
- Multiple comorbidities can alter blood glucose independent of a diagnosis of diabetes.

INTRODUCTION

With an estimated more than 100 million people in the United States living with prediabetes or diabetes, practitioners in all disciplines need to have a clear understanding of the criteria for diagnosing a patient with diabetes.[1] Practitioners need to know the history behind the current guidelines, the various diagnostic tests available, diagnostic criteria for diabetes, and a few rare but clinically relevant conditions that have an impact on blood sugar.

The American Diabetes Association (ADA) is leading "the fight against the deadly consequences of diabetes and fight[s] for those affected by diabetes."[2] Founded in 1939, the ADA seeks to provide research funding, community services, and training materials for patients, families, and medical providers. Each year, the ADA releases

[a] PA Online Program, Yale University, 100 Church Street South, Suite A230, Room A235, PO Box 208004, New Haven, CT 06520-8004, USA; [b] Neighborhood Outreach Access to Health - HonorHealth, 9201 North 5th Street, Phoenix, AZ 85020, USA
* Corresponding author.
E-mail address: stephanie.neary@yale.edu

Physician Assist Clin 5 (2020) 109–120
https://doi.org/10.1016/j.cpha.2019.11.012
2405-7991/20/© 2019 Elsevier Inc. All rights reserved.

physicianassistant.theclinics.com

updates to the "Standards of Medical Care in Diabetes,"[3] an evidence-based guideline for providing up-to-date, comprehensive care to patients with diabetes. There is even an abridged version specifically for primary care providers.

WHEN TO SCREEN FOR DIABETES

Although diabetes is prevalent throughout the United States, not all individuals need be tested; there are clear guidelines in place for who should be screened and when screening should take place (**Figs. 1** and **2**).

An elevated hemoglobin A_{1c} (HbA_{1c}) should be repeated to confirm diagnosis except in patients with unequivocal hyperglycemia. The fasting plasma glucose (FPG) test and oral glucose tolerance test (OGTT) require either two abnormal values separated temporally, or abnormal values on two different diagnostic tests run from the same sample (**Table 1**). Random plasma glucose (RPG) test is only diagnostic if a patient also has clinical symptoms of hyperglycemia (ie, polydipsia, polyuria, and unexplained weight loss) or symptoms of a hyperglycemic crisis. If there are large discrepancies between HbA_{1c} and these testing results, the patient should be screened for conditions that can have an impact on the accuracy of HbA_{1c} testing, such as sickle cell anemia (**Table 2**).

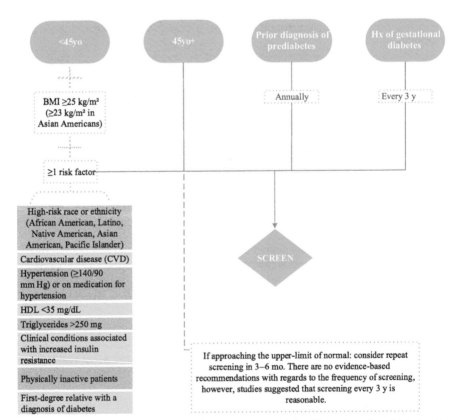

Fig. 1. Asymptomatic patients: criteria for screening in adults. (*From* American Diabetes Association. Standards of Medical Care in Diabetes—2019 Abridged for Primary Care Providers. (2018). *Clin Diabetes.* 2019 Jan;37(1):11-34.)

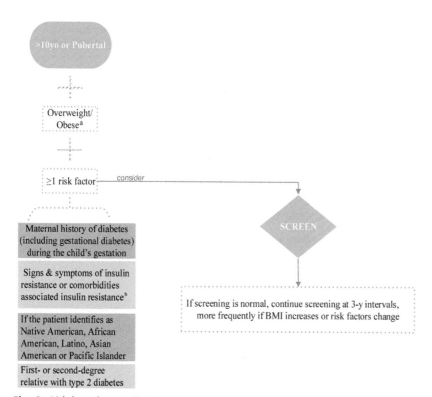

Fig. 2. Risk-based screening in asymptomatic children and adolescents. [a] Overweight = ≥85%ile, obese = ≥95%ile. [b] Signs and symptoms include polyuria, polydipsia, polyphagia, acanthosis nigricans; comorbidities include hypertension, hyperlipidemia, PCOS. (*From* American Diabetes Association. Standards of Medical Care in Diabetes—2019 Abridged for Primary Care Providers. (2018). *Clin Diabetes.* 2019 Jan;37(1):11-34.)

There are many laboratory tests available to screen for diabetes

Hemoglobin A₁c

- Also called A_{1c}, HbA_{1c}, or glycated hemoglobin

- Measures the amount of hemoglobin A (accounts for 90% of total hemoglobin) with bound glucose (glycated) and is reported as a percentage, with a higher percentage indicating more severe disease

- Serves as an approximately 3-month average of glucose due to rate of red blood cell turnover; HbA_{1c} is less sensitive than glucose testing to acute changes in carbohydrate intake, stress, or illness
  - Point-of-care HbA_{1c} testing can only be used for monitoring, not diagnosis.

- Results
  - Normal: ≤5.6%
  - Prediabetes: 5.7%–6.4%
  - Diabetes: ≥6.5%

- Limitations
  - Lower sensitivity than glucose testing
  - Unreliable in patients with certain comorbidities (see **Table 2**)

Fasting plasma glucose

- Requires 8 hours of fasting (water is permissible) prior to blood glucose testing.
  - Blood glucose testing is required for diagnosis; point-of-care meter testing can be used for monitoring only.
- Results
  - Normal: less than 100 mg/dL
  - Prediabetes: 100 mg/dL–125 mg/dL
  - Diabetes: ≥126 mg/dL
- Limitations
  - Limited to current glucose levels that are highly sensitive to changes due to recent carbohydrate intake, stress, or illness
  - Less correlation to long-term complications of diabetes than HbA$_{1c}$
  - Many laboratory tests wrongfully test serum glucose

Oral glucose tolerance testing

- Requires 8 hours of fasting (water is permissible) prior to testing
  - Procedure
    - Baseline fasting blood glucose test
    - Patient drinks oral glucose drink, 75 g, in a 5-min period
    - Two hours later, blood glucose levels tested again
- Results (at 2 hours post 75-g glucose load)
  - Normal: less than 139 mg/dL
  - Prediabetes: 140 mg/dL–199 mg/dL
  - Diabetes: ≥200 mg/dL
- Limitations
  - Impacted by acute changes in stress, illness, or medications; caffeine consumption; or tobacco use

IF HEMOGLOBIN A$_{1c}$ IS NOT RELIABLE, WHAT CAN BE DONE?

Fructosamine and glycated albumin (GA) testing offer potential solutions for monitoring glucose control in the presence of hemoglobinopathies.[4] Much like HbA$_{1c}$ measures glycated hemoglobin, fructosamine testing measures glycated protein, which includes albumin plus glycated lipoproteins and glycated globulins; GA testing measures GA alone.

Fructosamine and GA are predictive of blood sugars only over the 2 to 3 weeks prior to testing, compared with a period of 2 months to 3 months prior to testing with HbA1c testing, a feature that can be beneficial when looking at more rapidly changing metabolic states. Because albumin and other plasma proteins are more sensitive to glycation than hemoglobin, both fructosamine and GA testing reflect changes in blood sugar more rapidly than HbA$_{1c}$ (**Table 3**).

Table 1
Prediabetes and diabetes diagnostic criteria

Test	Prediabetes	Diabetes
HbA$_{1c}$	5.7%–6.4%	≥6.5%
FPG	100–125 mg/dL	≥126 mg/dL
OGTT	140–199 mg/dL	≥200 mg/dL
RPG		≥200 mg/dL

Data from American Diabetes Association. Standards of Medical Care in Diabetes—2019 Abridged for Primary Care Providers. (2018). *Clin Diabetes.* 2019 Jan;37(1):11-34.

Table 2
Common situations that make hemoglobin A$_{1c}$ less reliable

Factors Associated with False Levels	Why Hemoglobin A$_{1c}$ is Impacted
False decrease ↓	
Antiretroviral treatment of HIV	Causes low hemolytic state that shortens RBC life span
Blood transfusions	New RBCs in circulation
Chronic liver disease	Bleeding and hemolysis shorten RBC life span
Hemodialysis	Shortened life span of RBC
Erythropoietin treatment	New RBCs in circulation
Hemolytic anemia	Shortened life span of RBC
High-dose vitamin C or vitamin E supplementation	Inhibition of glycation
Sickle cell anemia	Presence of HbF causes assay artifact
Thalassemia	HB S-beta causes shortened RBC life span
False increase ↑	
Anemia: iron deficiency, vitamin B$_{12}$ deficiency, folate deficiency, and aplastic	Increased life span of RBC
Chronic kidney disease without dialysis	Increase in glycation
Splenectomy	Increased life span of RBC

Abbreviations: Hb, Hemoglobin; HbF, fetal hemoglobin; HIV, human immunodeficiency virus; RBC, red blood cell.

Adapted from Pippitt K, Li M, Gurgle HE. Diabetes Mellitus: Screening and Diagnosis. Am Fam Physician. 2016 Jan 15;93(2):103-9.

Table 3
Alternate screening tests

Test	Description	When to Order	Notes
C peptide	Predictive of endogenous insulin production as preproinsulin → proinsulin → insulin + C peptide C peptide is easier to measure in the blood than insulin.	• Suspect LADA • Suspect T1DM but autoantibodies are negative • After pancreatic surgery • Suspect insulinoma	Blood glucose must be measured at time of testing to ensure proper stimulation of insulin production.
Anti-GAD	Presence of GAD antibodies are associated with the development of T1DM and LADA	• Adult who does not have risk factors associated with diabetes • Patient with T2DM with decreased sensitivity to oral medications • Suspected T1DM during pregnancy	

Also consider ordering islet cell cytoplasmic autoantibodies, IA-2 autoantibodies, and insulin autoantibodies.

These tests are not without limitation. Unfortunately, fructosamine and GA tests lack standardization of results and thus are unable to be utilized for diagnostic purposes. Monitoring trends in levels over time can be useful in determining the efficacy of medication management, but no clear guidelines for insulin titration based on fructosamine or GA levels currently exist. Both tests, in the presence of any condition that has an impact on serum albumin (such as hepatic or kidney disease), can be unreliable.

DIABETES CLASSIFICATIONS
Prediabetes

Prediabetes is a high-risk state in which glucose levels are greater than normal and may continue to increase, thus approaching diabetic levels.[5] Prediabetes is defined as the presence of impaired fasting glucose, impaired glucose tolerance (IGT), and/or the diagnostic values discussed later (**Table 4**).

Table 4 Diagnostic criteria for prediabetes	
Prediabetes	
HbA_{1c}	5.7%–6.4%
FPG	100–125 mg/dL
OGTT	140–199 mg/dL

Data from American Diabetes Association. Standards of Medical Care in Diabetes—2019 Abridged for Primary Care Providers. Clin Diabetes. 2019 Jan;37(1):11-34.

Type 1 Diabetes Mellitus

Type 1 diabetes mellitus (T1DM) can be subdivided into immune-mediated diabetes and idiopathic diabetes.

Immune-mediated diabetes is defined by the presence of at least 1 of the following autoantibodies:

1. Islet cell autoantibodies
2. Autoantibodies to insulin
3. Autoantibodies to Glutamic acid decarboxylase (GAD_{65}) antibodies
4. Autoantibodies to the tyrosine phosphatases IA-2 and IA-2B
5. Autoantibodies to zinc transporter 8

Additionally, there is a known HLA association between immune-mediated diabetes and the DQA and DQB genes, which has proved to be either predisposing or protective, depending on the individual. C peptide also is a helpful test to measure progression of β-cell dysfunction because levels decrease with disease progression, indicating decreasing insulin production.

Idiopathic diabetes has no known etiology and cannot be attributed to an immune-mediated response. Individuals with idiopathic diabetes do not have autoantibodies present but do develop episodic ketoacidosis and have highly varied levels of β-cell function. Idiopathic diabetes typically is inherited and is not HLA associated.[6]

Type 2 Diabetes Mellitus

Type 2 diabetes mellitus (T2DM) is diagnosed either by hemoglobin A_1c, fasting plasma glucose, oral glucose tolerance testing, or random plasma glucose (**Table 5 and 6**)

Table 5
Type 2 diabetes mellitus diagnostic criteria

HbA$_{1c}$	≥6.5%
FPG	≥126 mg/dL
OGTT	≥200 mg/dL
RPG test	≥200 mg/dL

Data from American Diabetes Association. Classification and Diagnosis of Diabetes: Standards of Medical Care in Diabetes-2019. *Diabetes Care.* 2019 Jan;42(Suppl 1):S13-S28. https://doi.org/10.2337/dc19-S002.

Table 6
Diagnostic considerations for diabetes

Factors	Type 1 Diabetes Mellitus	Type 2 Diabetes Mellitus	Latent Autoimmune Diabetes in Adults
Age, y	<35	>35	>30
C peptide	Very low	Normal to high	Moderately low
Autoantibodies	At least 1 present	Not present	At least 1 present
Insulin requirement	At onset	Possibly with progression	Typically, within 6 mo

This table summarizes frequent trends in diabetes diagnostics; independently, these cannot be used to diagnose diabetes.

American Diabetes Association. Classification and Diagnosis of Diabetes: Standards of Medical Care in Diabetes-2018. *Diabetes Care.* 2018 Jan;41(Suppl 1):S13-S27.

Gestational diabetes

ADA guidelines state that all pregnant women should be screened for undiagnosed diabetes at their first prenatal visit and again at 24-weeks' gestation for gestational diabetes mellitus (GDM).[3] There are both 1-step and 2-step methods for diagnosing GDM (**Table 7**).

Table 7
One-step oral glucose tolerance test criteria

Fasting	≥92 mg/dL
1 h	≥180 mg/dL
2 h	≥153 mg/dL

American Diabetes Association. Classification and Diagnosis of Diabetes: Standards of Medical cAre in Diabetes-2019. *Diabetes Care.* 2019 Jan;42(Suppl 1):S13-S28. https://doi.org/10.2337/dc19-S002.

One-step testing

Between 24 weeks' and 28 weeks' gestation, after fasting for greater than or equal to 8 hours, give glucose oral load, 75 g. GDM can be diagnosed if any of the following plasma glucose values are met (**Table 7**).

Two-step

Step 1: The first step occurs between 24 weeks' and 28 weeks' gestation, when the patient is not fasting, give oral glucose load, 50 g. If the plasma glucose at 1 hour is greater than or equal to 130 mg/dL, proceed to step 2.

Table 8	
Two-step oral glucose tolerance test criteria	
Fasting	≥105 mg/dL
1 h	≥190 mg/dL
2 h	≥165 mg/dL
3 h	≥145 mg/dL

American Diabetes Association. Classification and Diagnosis of Diabetes: Standards of Medical cAre in Diabetes-2019. *Diabetes Care*. 2019 Jan;42(Suppl 1):S13-S28. https://doi.org/10.2337/dc19-S002.

Step 2: The second step is performed after fasting for greater than or equal to 8 hours, give oral glucose load, 100 g. GDM can be diagnosed if greater than or equal to 2 of the following plasma glucose levels are met (**Table 8**).

Diagnostic criteria and plasma value cutoff recommendations vary slightly between the ADA, National Diabetes Data Group, and American College of Obstetricians and Gynecologists. The numbers used in **Table 8** are from the National Diabetes Data Group and supported by the ADA.[6]

Sometimes, It Is a Zebra

Although a vast majority of patients with diabetes fit into the well-defined categories of T1DM, T2DM, or GDM, there are a few other, less common diagnoses that cannot be overlooked.

Latent autoimmune diabetes in adults

Latent autoimmune diabetes in adults (LADA) often is misdiagnosed and treated as T2DM due to the mixed clinical features between T1DM and T2DM. Patients with LADA have decreased β-cell function, as evidenced by decreased C-peptide levels, but not as low as seen with T1DM. Additionally, due to the autoimmune nature of the condition, at least 1 of the following autoantibodies is present, as also is the case with T1DM:

1. Islet cell autoantibodies
2. Autoantibodies to insulin
3. Autoantibodies to glutamic acid decarboxylase (GAD_{65}) antibodies
4. Autoantibodies to the tyrosine phosphatases IA-2 and IA-2B
5. Autoantibodies to zinc transporter 8

clinical pearl: patients who are above age 30 at the onset of diabetes, have a normal body mass index, and appear to be resistant to oral medications should be screened for LADA because they do not fit the clinical picture of or have the medication response expected of T2DM.

Monogenic diabetes

In rare situations, decreased insulin production can be linked to a single, usually inherited gene defect. This is significantly different from the combination of polygenic inheritance and environmental factors seen with both T1DM and T2DM. Monogenic diabetes should be considered in all patients where any of the following clinical factors is present:

- Diagnosis occurs at ≤6 months of life.
- Comorbidities are caused by other specific gene mutations (ie, polycystic kidney disease).

- Nonobese (BMI < 30) patients with family members who have diabetes
- Having a parent with any type of diabetes

The two most common types of monogenic diabetes are maturity-onset diabetes of the young (MODY) and neonatal diabetes mellitus (NDM).

Maturity-onset diabetes of the young MODY is an inherited (autosomal dominant) form of diabetes that accounts for 1% to 2% of all patients with diabetes.[7] Typically, patients with MODY present with subacute ketosis, a key differentiating factor for T1DM patients. Patients are nonobese and without the comorbidities often present in patients with T2DM. There currently are greater than 9 identified genetic mutations that can result in the MODY phenotype. Not all patients require insulin for glucose regulation.

MODY can be differentiated from T1DM because C peptide remains normal and GAD antibodies are negative

Neonatal diabetes mellitus Diabetes with onset before 6 months to 12 months of life almost always is due to an identifiable genetic cause.[8] Infants with NDM do not produce enough insulin, resulting in elevated blood glucose levels. NDM can be further categorized, with a close to even divide, into permanent NDM and transient NDM. Permanent NDM is a lifelong condition whereas patients with transient NDM typically have a resolution of symptoms during infancy but potential reappearance as they age. NDM also should be suspected with intrauterine growth restriction and failure to thrive.

Diagnosis: Genetic testing is required to diagnose NDM.

Steroid-induced hyperglycemia

Glucocorticoids frequently are prescribed for a wide variety of medical conditions, both short term and long term in duration.[9] The effect on blood glucose depends highly on the steroid medication type, the dose given, and the frequency of administration. Intermediate-acting steroids (methylprednisolone and prednisone) peak at 4 hours to 6 hours, causing afternoon hyperglycemia when given in a single morning dose. Long-acting steroids (dexamethasone) can cause persistent hyperglycemia for 24 hours or longer. In very high doses, as seen with chemotherapy treatments, dexamethasone can cause elevated blood sugars for multiple days after administration. Incidence of steroid-induced hyperglycemia in patients without a prior history ranges from 34.3% to 56%. Diagnosis is consistent with ADA guidelines for diabetes, with the specifier of steroid-induced rather than type 1 or type 2. All patients beginning steroid therapy should have a baseline blood glucose test and be taught how to properly monitor their glucose levels at home as well as the symptoms of both hyperosmolar hyperglycemic state and hypoglycemia (**Box 1**).

There is minimal or no known risk of hyperglycemia as a result of glucocorticoid-containing inhalers, topical preparations, or eye drops.

Stress-induced hyperglycemia

There currently are no set diagnostic criteria for stress-induced hyperglycemia.[10] Any persistent elevation in glucose in a person with no prior history of diabetes who is undergoing surgery or another stress-inducing medical event can be classified as stress-induced hyperglycemia. It is estimated that 30% of Americans are unaware of their current diabetes or prediabetes diagnosis. For patients with a history of diabetes or those undergoing procedures that carry a risk of postoperative hyperglycemia, such as transplant procedures, some orthopedic procedures, and gastric bypass procedures, many hospital systems order an HbA_{1c} prior to surgery

---

Box 1
Case 1: a newly diagnosed patient

Ms A is a 37-year-old woman who presented to the emergency department (ED) with a blood glucose of 39 mg/dL. She reports that 6 weeks ago she was diagnosed with T2DM (HbA$_{1c}$: 7.5%) while hospitalized for her third round of chemotherapy for stage IV endometrial cancer. She reports no prior history of prediabetes/diabetes. After her diagnosis, she followed-up with her primary care provider (PCP) and was prescribed metformin, 1000 mg twice a day, and insulin glargine (Lantus), 15 units twice a day, and instructed to follow-up in 3 months for HbA$_{1c}$ testing. Ms A received her fourth round of chemotherapy 9 days prior to her current ER visit, which included high-dose dexamethasone on each of the 2 days preceding treatment and the 2 days after treatment. Ms A reports her blood sugars spiked to 625 mg/dL, for which she gave herself 50 units of insulin glargine (Lantus) and arrived at the ED later that day with a glucose of 39 mg/dL.

Discussion: Ms A's HbA$_{1c}$ likely is elevated due to the high-dose steroids administered with each round of chemotherapy during the prior months, yet she was diagnosed with T2DM. Although she reports very high blood sugars for the 2 weeks after her chemotherapy, she reports normal sugars for the remainder of the month until her next round begins. A fixed, long-acting insulin regimen does not accommodate for the lasting impact of steroids on her blood glucose, causing highly varied levels throughout the month.

Plan: Ms A was discharged on 2 separate insulin regimens

For the 2 weeks after chemotherapy
- Insulin glargine (Lantus), 30 units every night at bedtime
- Regular insulin 3ac (before meals)
- Sliding scale regular insulin (sliding scale insulin before meals according to scale: 150–179 mg/dL: 3 units; 180–229 mg/dL: 6 units; 230–279 mg/dL: 9 units; 280–329 mg/dL: 12 units; 330–379 mg/dL: 15 units; and >380 mg/dL: 18 units; and sliding scale insulin at bedtime according to scale: 200–229 mg/dL: 3 units; 230–279 mg/dL: 6 units; 280–329 mg/dL: 9 units; 330–379 mg/dL: 12 units; and >380 mg/dL: 15 units)

And for the other 2 weeks
- Insulin glargine (Lantus), 20 units every night at bedtime
- Regular insulin 3ac (before meals)
- Sliding scale with regular insulin (sliding scale insulin with meals according to scale: 150–179 mg/dL: 1 unit; 180–229 mg/dL: 2 units; 230–279 mg/dL: 3 units; 280–329 mg/dL: 4 units; 330–379 mg/dL: 5 units; and >380 mg/dL: 6 units; and sliding scale insulin at bedtime according to scale: 200–229 mg/dL: 1 unit; 230–279 mg/dL: 2 units; 280–329 mg/dL: 3 units; 330–379 mg/dL: 4 units; and >380 mg/dL: 5 units)[a]

Ms. A met with a Certified Diabetes Educator and a registered dietician before discharge to discuss sliding scale insulin and dangers of self-determined titration without provider guidance.

[a] Regular insulin was selected over insulin aspart for mealtime and sliding scale regular insulin due to cost because patient is currently uninsured.

Data from Dungan KM, Braithwaite SS, Preiser JC. Stress hyperglycaemia. *Lancet.* 2009 May 23;373(9677):1798-807.

---

to establish a baseline but, in emergent situations, this often is not possible. Typically, as a patient recovers from the stress-inducing event, blood sugars begin to return to normal. If sugars remain elevated, it is prudent to explore other possible classifications of diabetes.

Conditions associated with hyperglycemia
Hereditary hemochromatosis Hereditary hemochromatosis is caused by a defect in the HFE gene, which results in increased iron storage.[11] These iron deposits are

found in many organs, including the pancreas. There is an increased incidence of diabetes in individuals with hereditary hemochromatosis, but exact etiology remains unclear. Increased iron deposits in the skin can result in a darkening of skin tone, and, when paired with insulin resistance, sometimes has resulted in hemochromatosis referred to as bronze diabetes. Genetic testing is necessary for diagnosis and often is paired with iron panels and liver function tests.

Pancreatic cancer Currently, there is conflicting evidence on whether T2DM and insulin resistance are risk factors for or are caused by pancreatic cancer.[12] Although the direction of the association has not been clearly established, there is a clear correlation between individuals with T2DM and pancreatic cancer. Pancreatic cancer should be considered in the differential diagnosis for any patient with new-onset diabetes who does not fit the typical clinical picture of a patient with T2DM. Diagnosis of pancreatic cancer typically begins with imaging (ultrasound or CT scan) but requires biopsy for definitive diagnosis.

Cushing's syndrome A chronic hypercortisol state leads to increased insulin resistance and decreased insulin production.[13] The prevalence of IGT in patients with hypercortisolism is 27% compared with only 10% in matched controls. Hypercortisol-induced hyperglycemia should be diagnosed using the same glucose ranges as T2DM (**Table 6**) and is managed similarly.

Cystic fibrosis The most common comorbidity in patients with cystic fibrosis is cystic fibrosis–related diabetes (CFRD), affecting approximately 40% to 50% of adults and 20% of adolescents.[14] Hyperglycemia is caused by insulin insufficiency and often compounded by insulin resistance secondary to infection and inflammation. The ADA currently recommends annual screening for CFRD with OGTT starting at 10 years old if not previously diagnosed with CFRD. HbA$_{1c}$ is not recommended for screening or diagnosis.

Polycystic ovarian syndrome Insulin resistance occurs in 50% to 80% of women with polycystic ovarian syndrome (PCOS). Incidences of ICT and T2DM are reported at 31.3% and 7.1% of women, respectively, which is significantly higher than age-matched and weight-matched women without PCOS.[15] OGTT is considered the most accurate method for diagnosing IGT or T2DM in patients with PCOS and it is recommended that all women with PCOS be screened. Additionally, any new-onset diabetes in a patient who meets the clinical picture of a patient with PCOS (hirsutism, obesity, and abnormal menstruation) should be screened for PCOS.

SUMMARY

Despite the vast majority of patients diagnosed with diabetes in the United States being classified as either T1DM or T2DM, increased understanding of the pathophysiology of diabetes has provided insight to the complexity of properly diagnosing a patient who presents with hyperglycemia. There are multiple considerations when navigating a diagnosis of diabetes, a field that continues to grow with emerging research.

DISCLOSURE

The authors have nothing to disclose.

REFERENCES

1. National Center for Chronic Disease Prevention and Health Promotion: Division of diabetes translation. National diabetes statistics report, 2017: estimates of diabetes and its burden in the United States. 2017. Available at: https://www.cdc.gov/diabetes/pdfs/data/statistics/national-diabetes-statistics-report.pdf. Accessed May 15, 2019.
2. American Diabetes Association: about us. Available at: http://www.diabetes.org/about-us/. Accessed May 15, 2019.
3. American Diabetes Association. Classification and diagnosis of diabetes: standards of medical care in diabetes-2019. Diabetes Care 2019;42(Suppl 1): S13–28.
4. Danese E, Montagnana M, Nouvenne A, et al. Advantages and pitfalls of fructosamine and glycated albumin in the diagnosis and treatment of diabetes. J Diabetes Sci Technol 2015;9(2):169–76.
5. American Diabetes Association. Standards of medical care in diabetes—2019 abridged for primary care providers. Clin Diabetes 2019;37(1):11–34.
6. American Diabetes Association. Classification and diagnosis of diabetes: standards of medical care in diabetes-2018. Diabetes Care 2018;41(Suppl 1): S13–27.
7. Juszczak A, Pryse R, Schuman A, et al. When to consider a diagnosis of MODY at the presentation of diabetes: aetiology matters for correct management. Br J Gen Pract 2016;66(647):e457–9.
8. Rudland VL. Diagnosis and management of glucokinase monogenic diabetes in pregnancy: current perspectives. Diabetes Metab Syndr Obes 2019;12:1081–9.
9. Tamez-Pérez HE, Quintanilla-Flores DL, Rodriquez-Gutierrez R, et al. Steroid hyperglycemia: Prevalence, early detection and therapeutic recommendations: a narrative review. World J Diabetes 2015;6(8):1073–81.
10. Dungan KM, Braithwaite SS, Preiser JC. Stress hyperglycaemia. Lancet 2009; 373(9677):1798–807.
11. Franchini M, Veneri D. Recent advances in hereditary hemochromatosis. Ann Hematol 2005;84(6):347–52.
12. De Souza A, Irfan K, Masud F, et al. Diabetes type 2 and pancreatic cancer: a history unfolding. JOP 2016;17(2):144–8.
13. Colao A, De Block C, Gaztambide MS, et al. Managing hyperglycemia in patients with Cushing's disease treated with pasireotide: medical expert recommendations. Pituitary 2014;17(2):180–6.
14. Kelsey R, Manderson Koivula FN, McClenaghan NH, et al. Cystic fibrosis-related diabetes: pathophysiology and therapeutic challenges. Clin Med Insights Endocrinol Diabetes 2019;12. 11795514198517701.
15. Dumitrescu R, Mehedintu C, Briceag I, et al. The polycystic ovary syndrome: an update on metabolic and hormonal mechanisms. J Med Life 2015;8(2):142–5.

Ominous Octet and Other Scary Diabetes Stories
The Overview of Pathophysiology of Type 2 Diabetes Mellitus

Sarah Dion Kelly, MS, RD, CDE[a],*,
Stephanie L. Neary, MPA, MMS, PA-C[b]

KEYWORDS

- Type 2 diabetes • Pathophysiology of type 2 diabetes • Impaired glucose tolerance
- Insulin resistance • B cell dysfunction • Incretin hormone dysfunction

KEY POINTS

- Eight major shortfalls are identified as the primary causes of the pathophysiology of insulin resistance and type 2 diabetes.
- Insulin resistance in liver, muscle, and brain tissue coupled with failures in both α and β cell function within the pancreas are major pathophysiologic deficits seen in diabetes.
- Incretin hormone dysfunction and resistance fail to stimulate insulin release from the pancreas.
- Changes in lipolysis lead to excessive free fatty acid release and subsequent lipotoxicity, which further impair insulin secretion.
- In the kidneys, the set point for glucosuria increases with rising blood glucose leading to further exacerbation of hyperglycemia.

INTRODUCTION

Type 2 diabetes (T2DM) has long been identified as a complex disease developing along a spectrum of metabolic and hormonal dysfunction occurring within the context of genetic and environmental influences. It is now well accepted that impaired fasting glucose (IFG), impaired glucose tolerance (IGT), and prediabetes precede the development of T2DM. Early screening and diagnosis in at-risk populations offer opportunities to delay progression of disease and improve long-term treatment outcomes. Understanding the complex pathophysiologic causes of T2DM helps clinicians provide multifaceted approaches to therapeutic strategies.

[a] Inova Center for Wellness and Metabolic Health, 2740 Prosperity Avenue, Suite 200, Fairfax, VA 22031, USA; [b] Yale University Physician Assistant Online Program, 100 Church Street South, Suite A230, Room A235, New Haven, CT 06520, USA
* Corresponding author. PO Box 208004, New Haven, CT 06520-8004.
E-mail address: Sarah.kelly@yale.edu

Physician Assist Clin 5 (2020) 121–133
https://doi.org/10.1016/j.cpha.2019.11.002
2405-7991/20/© 2020 Elsevier Inc. All rights reserved.

Eight major shortfalls are identified as the primary causes of the pathophysiology of insulin resistance and T2DM. DeFronzo[1] first described this "Ominous Octet" in 2009. This expanded his previously described "triumvirate" approach to the pathogenesis of T2DM, which identified only 3 major shortfalls: insulin resistance in the muscle, insulin resistance in the liver, and β cell failure.[2] There is an interplay in the pathophysiologic dysfunction seen in T2DM among multiple organ systems throughout the body. The ominous octet involves major deficits observed in the liver, brain, muscle tissue, adipose tissue, kidneys, gastrointestinal (GI) tract, and pancreas (**Fig. 1, Box 1**).

T2DM develops along a spectrum, marked initially by hyperinsulinemia with normal glucose levels followed by hyperinsulinemia with concomitant hyperglycemia.[3] Eventually β cell failure and insulin deficiency result in frank hyperglycemia. Prediabetes and diabetes diagnostic criteria are listed in **Table 1**.[3]

IFG is more often seen in men, whereas IGT is more often apparent in women.[4] Overt diabetes develops when pancreatic β cell function falls to less than 50%.[1,5] Beta cell failure occurs along a timeline of unknown length involving an interplay between genetic predisposition and environmental and lifestyle influences. Multiple common risk variants related to T2DM are identified in genome-wide association studies, and these variants are associated with diabetes-related metabolite traits.[6] Environmental and lifestyle influences include but are not limited to age, sex, dietary intake, obesity, physical inactivity, socioeconomic status, and stress level.[3] Dimorphic differences exist among risk factors and pathogenesis of diabetes.[4] "Metabolic memory" explores the concept that patients who achieve glycemic control early in the natural history of their disease may reduce their risk of long-term complications in comparison with those that have years of suboptimal glycemic control.[7,8] It is clear that early and intensive interventions reduce complications and help patients toward better long-term outcomes.[7,8]

INSULIN RESISTANCE: LIVER, MUSCLE, BRAIN, ADIPOSE TISSUE

Insulin resistance is a hallmark feature of T2DM and is observed most notably in liver, muscle, brain, and adipose tissue. In the patient with T2DM, insulin does not work appropriately at normal physiologic levels in these targeted tissues. Insulin is an anabolic hormone responsible for the activities listed in **Box 2**.

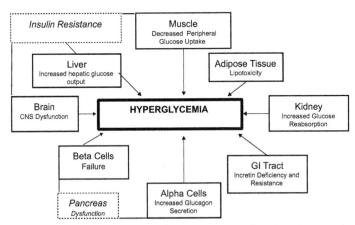

Fig. 1. The ominous octet. (*Data from* Defronzo RA. From the triumvirate to the ominous octet: a new paradigm for the treatment of type 2 diabetes mellitus. Diabetes Care 2009;58(4):773–95.)

> **Box 1**
> **The ominous octet**
>
> 1. Liver: insulin resistance and increased glucose production
> 2. Muscle: insulin resistance and reduced peripheral glucose uptake
> 3. Brain: insulin resistance and CNS dysfunction
> 4. Adipose tissue: insulin resistance, lipotoxicity, and proinflammatory markers
> 5. Kidneys: increased glucose production and reabsorption
> 6. GI tract: incretin hormone dysfunction and resistance
> 7. Pancreatic β cells: failure and dysfunction
> 8. Pancreatic α cells: hyperglucagonemia
>
> *Data from* DeFronzo RA. From the triumvirate to the ominous octet: a new paradigm for the treatment of type 2 diabetes mellitus. Diabetes 2009;58(4):773–95.

In the healthy liver, insulin encourages the uptake of glucose. It also inhibits gluconeogenesis through its effects on gene expression of the rate-limiting enzymes glucose-6-phosphatase, phosphoenolpyruvate (PEP) carboxylase, and fructose 1,6-bisphosphatase.[9] In healthy muscle, insulin increases the uptake of glucose through translocation of intracellular GLUT4 receptors to the surface of the cell, which in turn increases uptake of glucose, encouraging glycogen synthesis.[9] In adipose tissue, insulin suppresses lipolysis and encourages uptake of glucose into adipocytes for lipogenesis.[10] In the brain, insulin and other peripheral hormones regulate hepatic glucose production and appetite regulation.[11]

In T2DM, hepatocytes fail to regulate glucose production; muscle does not take up glucose efficiently, lipolysis is not suppressed, and central nervous system (CNS) dysfunction is manifested, leading to an inadequate regulation of appetite and metabolism.[10] Globally, hyperinsulinemia leads to a downregulation of insulin receptors on cell surfaces.[12] Peripheral and visceral fat deposition is a major contributing factor to insulin resistance.[13] White adipose tissue releases proinflammatory markers that influence insulin action.[14] These hallmark features summarize the pathophysiologic effects related to insulin resistance.

Liver

The liver maintains blood glucose levels within normal range during fasting states primarily through glycogenolysis (glycogen breakdown resulting in glucose release) and

Table 1
Prediabetes and diabetes diagnostic criteria

Test	Prediabetes	Diabetes
A1C	5.7%–6.4%	≥6.5%
FPG	100–125 mg/dL	≥126 mg/dL
OGTT	140–199 mg/dL	≥200 mg/dL
RPG		≥200 mg/dL

Abbreviations: A1C, hemoglobin A1c, glycated hemoglobin; FPG, fasting plasma glucose; OGTT, oral glucose tolerance test; RPG, random plasma glucose.
Data from American Diabetes Association. Standards of Medical Care in Diabetes—2019 Abridged for Primary Care Providers. (2018). Clin Diabetes. 2019 Jan;37(1):11–34.

> **Box 2**
> **Insulin is an anabolic hormone**
>
> 1. Regulation of both glucose production and storage
> 2. Glucose uptake in both liver and muscle
> 3. Suppression of lipolysis
> 4. Influence over metabolism and appetite in the CNS
>
> *Data from* Costanzo LS. Endocrine physiology. In: Physiology, 6e, Philadelphia: Elsevier; 2018: 395-460.

gluconeogenesis (glucose synthesis). Fasting hyperglycemia that occurs in T2DM is a result of increased hepatic glucose production via unchecked gluconeogenesis. A gradual loss in signaling factors, known as Forkhead Box Protein O (FoxO), that influence insulin action within the liver results from a breakdown in insulin's ability to suppress hepatic gluconeogenesis, specifically on the rate-limiting enzyme, glucose-6-phosphatase. FoxO factors are broadly described as a family of signaling transcription factors that direct insulin action in the liver.[15] FoxO also targets β cell transcription factors in the pancreas.[5] Pajani and Acilli[16,17] described FoxO as a key factor in maintaining "metabolic flexibility" with regard to hepatic glucose and lipid metabolism. Insulin, under the guidance of FoxO factors, directs the junction between glucose production and lipogenesis, specifically glucose-6-phosphatase (glucose production) and glucokinase (glucose/fat storage).[16,17] As insulin levels rise to suppress elevated glucose, glucose-6-phosphatase is inhibited to prevent gluconeogenesis. However, with hyperinsulinemia, FoxO signaling is inactivated and the suppression of glucose-6-phosphatase results in increased activation of glucokinase, leading to an increase in lipogenesis.[16] This results in increased free fatty acids in the liver, which feed gluconeogenesis, playing a key role in the pathogenesis of increased hepatic glucose production.[15,17]

Muscle

In muscle tissue, insulin resistance manifests as defects in intracellular phosphorylation and glucose transport.[18,19] Impairment in insulin access and signaling in the muscle microvasculature are responsible for these deficits.[19] In the muscle, insulin directly affects the action of hexokinase, glucose synthase, and pyruvate dehydrogenase and its deficit, either via insulin deficiency or because of resistance, reduces glycogen synthesis and glycolysis in the muscle cell, leaving plasma glucose levels to increase.[10]

Insulin modulates vascular tone and perfusion throughout the body by binding to insulin receptors and insulin-like growth factor receptors and by stimulating 2 different pathways: the phosphoinositide 3-kinase/phosphokinase B (PI3-kinase/PKB) pathway and the mitogen-activated protein kinase (MAPK) pathway.[10,19] The PI3-kinase/PKB pathway activates endothelial nitric oxide synthase, increasing the presence of nitric oxide, which induces a "heart healthy" state of vasodilation and reduces platelet and immune cell adhesion. The MAPK pathway activates secretion of endothelin-1 and induces an atherogenic state by increasing vasoconstriction, oxidative stress, and cell growth.[10,15]

In a healthy metabolic state, insulin balances these 2 pathways to stimulate glucose transport across the membrane of muscle cells. In a healthy state, insulin "tips the scale" via the PI3-kinase/PKB pathway, increasing vasodilation, which in turn relaxes muscle cell microvasculature and allows insulin to enter the muscle interstitium. This aids GLUT4 translocation and glucose transport into muscle cells.[19]

In the insulin-resistant state, the PI3-kinase/PKB pathway is impaired and the MAPK pathway dominates because of the influence of proinflammatory markers,[20] which include IκB kinase-β (IKKβ), c-Jun-N-terminal kinase 9 (JNK), and the nuclear factor (NF)-κB axis.[21] The MAPK pathway increases endothelin-1 release and subsequent vasoconstriction, reducing insulin's ability to enter muscle microvasculature, and prevents glucose uptake, exacerbating insulin resistance and hyperglycemia.[19] The excessive MAPK pathway stimulation also helps to describe the chronic atherogenic state that coincides with insulin resistance and T2DM.[19] **Fig. 2** is a depiction of these 2 opposing states.

Brain

The hypothalamus and pituitary gland coordinate numerous peripherally released hormones to influence appetite, energy balance, and metabolism.[10] Insulin, leptin, glucagon, GLP-1, and ghrelin influence glucose levels via the CNS[11] (**Table 2**). These hormones communicate with the hypothalamus through numerous mechanisms, including direct nutrient sensing in the gut.[11] Glucose crosses the blood-brain barrier and is the primary source of energy for neurons and glial cells. Glucose-excited neurons and glucose-inhibited neurons are present throughout the hypothalamus—specifically, the arcuate nucleus, ventromedial nucleus, dorsomedial nucleus, paraventricular nucleus, and lateral hypothalamus—to aid in regulation of glucose homeostasis.[11]

Insulin plays a key role in influencing hepatic and peripheral glucose as well as lipid metabolism via the CNS. In the healthy hypothalamus, insulin suppresses appetite.[10] Rodent studies of the hypothalamus have demonstrated that insulin acts to suppress hepatic glucose production,[22] encourages glucose uptake in muscle, and suppresses lipolysis.[23] Insulin activates the PI3-kinase/PKB pathway and K_{ATP} potassium channels in the neurons of the medial basal hypothalamus (MBH) as well as the MAPK pathway and K_{ATP} channels in the dorsal vagal complex (DVC), both resulting in a decrease in hepatic glucose production.[24,25]

Obesity is associated with CNS hormonal dysfunction. Overnutrition, high-fat feeding, and obesity promote insulin resistance in both the MBH and DVC, increasing hepatic glucose production and hyperphagia.[26] The ratio of cerebrospinal fluid insulin to plasma insulin is inversely related to body mass index (BMI), indicating potential problems with insulin transport into the hypothalamus as a cause of hypothalamic insulin resistance.[27,28] Proinflammatory markers seen in obesity, such as tumor necrosis

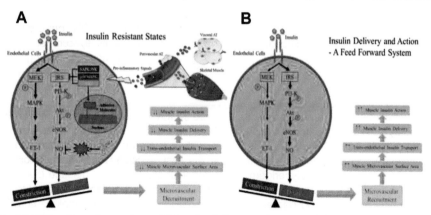

Fig. 2. (A) Insulin-resistant states. (B) Insulin delivery and actions. (*From* Liu J, Liu Z. Muscle insulin resistance and the inflamed microvasculature: fire from within. Int J Mol Sci 2019 Jan 29;20(3). pii: E562. https://doi.org/10.3390/ijms20030562; with permission.)

Table 2
Peripherally released hormones that influence glucose levels via CNS actions

Hormone	Origin	Function	Effect on Glucose
Insulin	Released from β cells of pancreas	Insulin is an anabolic hormone that is released in response to elevations in blood sugar and encourages glucose uptake in peripheral muscle, liver-stimulating glycogen synthesis, and lipogenesis	↓
Leptin	Released from adipocytes	Leptin influences energy balance and appetite in the hypothalamus	↓
Glucagon	Released from α cells of pancreas	Glucagon stimulates gluconeogenesis during periods of fasting	↓
GLP-1	Released from L cells of distal ileum	Incretin hormone released in response to meal to help lower blood sugar and stimulate insulin release	↓
CCK	Released from I cells of duodenum. Chyme entering the duodenum. May play a role in satiety signaling in the CNS	CCK is responsible for stimulating gallbladder contraction, and release of bile acids in response to chyme entering the duodenum. Also may play a role in satiety signaling in the CNS	↓
Ghrelin	Released by gastric cells	Ghrelin increases appetite and food intake	↑

Data from Costanzo LS. Gastrointestinal physiology. In: Physiology, 6e, Philadelphia: Elsevier, 2018: 339–393.

factor α (TNF-α), cause "hypothalamic inflammation" and induce insulin resistance similarly seen in other parts of the body via IKKβ and JNK pathways.[11]

Lastly, disturbances in the hypothalamic-pituitary-adrenal (HPA) axis and autonomic nervous system (ANS) can also be implicated in the pathogenesis of T2DM. Chronic overactivation of the HPA axis and ANS are seen in psychiatric diseases and neurodegenerative diseases, which have ties to metabolic syndrome, insulin resistance, and T2DM.[11]

Adipose Tissue

Manifestations in visceral adipose tissue, more so than in subcutaneous adipose tissue, play key roles in pathogenesis of T2DM. "Lipotoxicity" refers to the adverse effects of excessive circulating free fatty acids on insulin action and secretion. Lipotoxicity promotes insulin resistance in the liver, muscle, brain, and pancreas, and presents as hypertriglyceridemia and nonalcoholic fatty liver disease (NAFLD), common precipitating comorbidities for T2DM. In the liver, hyperinsulinemia inactivates FoxO signaling and decreases the glucose-6-phosphatase/glucokinase ratio, which also activates lipogenesis and leads to excessive free fatty acid production.[16] During insulin resistance, adipose tissue fails to regulate lipid metabolism, displays impaired mitochondrial function leading to anaerobic metabolism and lactate production, and generates proinflammatory markers, further exacerbating a chronic inflammatory state.[10,29]

BMI is well established as a leading risk factor for T2DM, with risk increasing 50- to 80-fold with BMI greater than 35.[13] Overnutrition, high-fat feeding, and obesity contribute to both subcutaneous and visceral fat stores. Location of ectopic fat deposition also determines the risk of insulin resistance in T2DM. Accumulation of adipose tissue perivascularly as well as in liver, muscle, and pancreas increases the risk of T2DM.[13]

Insulin plays an important role in lipid metabolism through suppression of lipolysis and stimulation of glucose uptake in adipocytes. Insulin receptors augment GLUT4 translocation to the adipocyte membrane via the insulin receptor cascade, stimulating the PI3-kinase/PKB pathway.[29] Glucose enters the adipocyte, glycolysis ensues, and glycerol-3-phosphate is produced. In turn, glycerol-3-phosphate provides the starting materials for lipogenesis. In the insulin-resistant state, insulin receptor activity and availability on the adipocyte are diminished, contributing to failure of 2 primary roles of adipose tissue: lipolysis during fasting and lipogenesis during feeding.[10] Among adipocytes, mitochondrial deficits are present owing to a decrease in the proteins necessary for proper β-oxidation.[30] This in turn leads to anaerobic metabolism and lactate production, resulting in a proinflammatory state.[29]

This accumulation of excess adipose tissue, specifically within visceral compartments, is associated with a proinflammatory state and a decreased presence of adiponectin.[31] Adiponectin is a hormone produced by adipocytes that aids in insulin sensitization, glucose homeostasis, and protection from inflammation.[32] Obesity increases the production of proinflammatory markers including TNF-α, interleukin (IL)-6, IL-1β, and IL-10.[14,21] These cytokines influence specific insulin signaling via IKKβ, JNK, and NF-κB and MAPK pathways, supporting inflammation, endoplasmic reticulum stress, and oxidative stress.[14] Chronic exposure, though not acute exposure, of IL-6 on adipocytes is associated with insulin resistance.[33]

KIDNEYS: INCREASED GLUCOSE PRODUCTION AND REABSORPTION

The kidneys have an impact on glucose homeostasis by way of three main functions as shown in **Box 3**. In the pathogenesis of T2DM, there are 2 manifestations observed in the kidneys: increased gluconeogenesis and increased glucose reabsorption.[34] These 2 shortcomings directly affect blood glucose levels and exacerbate hyperglycemia.

In the healthy kidney, postprandial and postabsorptive gluconeogenesis alongside what is produced in the liver accounts for a portion of usual glucose release. In addition, glucose is reabsorbed in the proximal convoluted tubule by a 2-step process: via active transport with sodium glucose cotransporters (SGLTs) followed by passive facilitated transport by GLUT transporters. This process is saturable.[35]

In T2DM, the kidneys inappropriately generate more glucose via gluconeogenesis, similarly to what is seen in the liver.[36] With regard to glucose reabsorption, as glucose levels increase in the blood, so does the threshold for glucose reabsorption.[37] It is unknown whether SGLT receptors upregulate in humans with T2DM or whether the tubules become hypertrophic and more efficient at reabsorbing glucose.[38] Typically, glucosuria is not observed in an individual without diabetes until blood glucose is ~200 mg/dL. However, in diabetes this threshold shifts and glucosuria may not be observed until 450 mg/dL. This efficient adaptation exacerbates hyperglycemia. **Fig. 3** demonstrates the glucose titration curve: as blood glucose levels increase, so does the threshold for glucose filtration, excretion, and reabsorption. The "splay"

Box 3
The kidneys affect glucose homeostasis by way of 3 main functions

1. Release glucose directly into the plasma by way of gluconeogenesis

2. Take up glucose from the circulation to meet energy needs

3. Reabsorb glucose from the glomerular filtrate, returning glucose to plasma circulation

Data from Gerich JE. Role of the kidney in normal glucose homeostasis and in the hyperglycae-mia of diabetes mellitus: therapeutic implications. Diabet Med 2010;27(2):136–42 and Alsahli M, Gerich JE. Renal glucose metabolism in normal physiology conditions and in diabetes. Diabetes Res Clin Pract 2017;133:1–9.

---

refers to heterogeneity in SGLT capability and subsequent differences in glucose threshold. Kidney glucose reabsorption is the target of SGLT inhibitors, a newer drug therapy for T2DM that efficiently addresses hyperglycemia, improves cardiovascular outcomes, and helps to preserve kidney function.[39]

GASTROINTESTINAL TRACT: INCRETIN DYSFUNCTION AND RESISTANCE

Incretin hormones include glucose-dependent insulinotropic polypeptide (GIP) and glucagon-like peptide-1 (GLP-1). These hormones are secreted in the gut and influence glucose homeostasis by enhancing insulin secretion from pancreatic β cells and suppressing glucagon secretion.[40] They also demonstrate additional effects in the body through influence on gastric emptying, intestinal transit time, appetite, food intake, energy balance, and lipid and bone metabolism.[40]

In the functioning GI tract, GIP is released from the K cells of the duodenum and upper jejunum and GLP-1 is released by the L cells throughout the small and large intestines in response to nutrient ingestion.[35] GIP and GLP-1 are secreted in response to carbohydrate intake more dramatically than protein or fat intake; all nutrients stimulate their release. As blood glucose levels increase after a meal, GIP and GLP-1 both bind to receptors on pancreatic β cells and enhance insulin secretion.[40]

Oral glucose ingestion, and the subsequent elevation in blood glucose, stimulates GIP and GLP-1 release more dramatically than intravenous glucose infusion, and this important phenomenon is known as the "incretin effect."[41] GIP and GLP-1 hormones may contribute between 25% and 75% of the insulin secretory response after an oral glucose load.[40] GLP-1 release also leads to a decrease in hepatic glucose production.[42]

Studies assessing GIP and GLP-1 in patients with T2DM have not consistently shown reduced secretion of these hormones in response to oral glucose tolerance tests and mixed meal tests when compared with healthy subjects.[43] However, there is evidence to support decreased incretin function and the possible development of incretin resistance in patients with T2DM, especially with long-standing disease.[43] Specifically, evidence in animal models exists to show decreased GLP-1 receptor function on β cells.[44] GLP-1 agonists now play an important therapeutic role in T2DM treatment strategies, and their use is associated with reduction in cardiovascular events and all-cause mortality.[45–47]

Dipeptidyl peptidase-4 (DPP-4) is a transmembrane proteolytic enzyme found in many types of cells throughout the body. DPP-4 plays a role in GLP-1 deactivation.[46] Higher circulatory DPP-4 levels and activity have been observed in a variety of metabolic diseases, including T2DM. DPP-4 inhibitors represent a newer pharmacologic strategy used to sustain the effects of GLP-1 by preventing their degradation.[47]

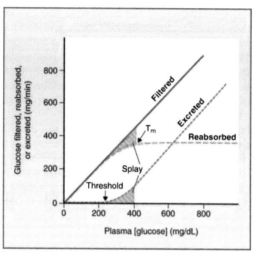

Fig. 3. Glucose titration curve. Glucose filtration, reabsorption, and excretion are shown as a function of plasma glucose concentration. Hatched areas represent the splay. T_m, tubular transport maximum. (*From* Costanzo LS. Chapter 6: Renal physiology. In: Physiology, sixth edition, pp. 245–310. Copyright 2018 by Elsevier, Inc.; reprinted with permission.)

PANCREAS

The pancreas serves both endocrine and exocrine secretory roles in the body. Exocrine acinar cells secrete digestive fluids into the duodenum and make up the majority of pancreatic mass.[48] There are 4 major types of hormone-secreting cells within the endocrine pancreas:

- α cells secrete glucagon
- β cells secrete insulin and amylin
- δ cells secrete somatostatin
- PP cells secrete pancreatic polypeptide[49]

These hormone-secreting cells cluster together into islets, known as islets of Langerhans. In the simplest terms, insulin lowers glucose levels and promotes glucose uptake and storage in peripheral tissues. Glucagon increases blood glucose levels through the stimulation of gluconeogenesis and subsequent release of glucose from both liver and kidney. Insulin is released from β cells via granule exocytosis once glucose enters the β cell by way of increased intracellular calcium and closure of K_{ATP} channels.[50] As mentioned earlier, GIP and GLP-1 hormones also bind to receptors on β cells to augment insulin secretion in the setting of hyperglycemia.[40]

Beta Cell Dysfunction and Failure

In the healthy pancreas, many signaling factors play important roles in β cell function and homeostasis and are targets for research. FoxO maintains β cell function via stimulation of 3 key transcription factors: pancreatic duodenal homeobox 1 (Pdx-1), NK6 homeobox 1 (NKx6.1), and musculoaponeurotic fibrosarcoma oncogene family A (MafA). Also, the Notch signaling pathway, initially thought to only direct differentiation during embryogenesis, now is known to aid in maintaining cell homeostasis in the adult β cell.[51] In the setting of metabolic stress, Pdx-1, NKx6.1, and MafA maintain β cell function and differentiation.[52–54] Hyperglycemia and dyslipidemia reduce the expression of these key regulating transcription factors and lead to "dedifferentiation" of the β cell or regression in their functional status.[5] In the setting of overnutrition and obesity, increased metabolic demands lead to stress and exhaustion on endoplasmic reticulum within β cells. Chronic β cell Notch signaling activation impairs glucose-stimulated insulin secretion in human islet cell and mouse models.[55] Over time, stressed β cells may dedifferentiate to α cells and produce glucagon, further exacerbating hyperglycemia and continuing to apoptosis.[5]

Differences in total pancreas mass and β cell mass are observed in obesity and T2DM. Obesity is associated with increases in total pancreas mass resulting from increased visceral adiposity. Decreased β cell mass, secondary to β cell death, is observed with long-standing T2DM.[48] Pancreatic islet cells are supported by an intricate network of endothelium that run along the capillary supply and are subject to oxidative stress and inflammation, leading to dysfunction in T2DM.[56]

Alpha Cells: Glucagonemia

Glucagon is released by α cells in the pancreas and its secretion is regulated by glucose levels. In the healthy pancreas, when glucose levels are low, glucagon is secreted because of the absence of insulin. Glucagon is released into the portal vein and stimulates gluconeogenesis and glucose release from the liver.[57,58] Insulin, somatostatin, and GLP-1 are released in response to hyperglycemia and suppress glucagon via paracrine signaling.[58] In patients with T2DM, high glucagon levels are observed throughout the day even with hyperglycemia.[59] These high levels of glucagon chronically stimulate glucose-6-phosphatase, which fuels increased hepatic glucose production and hyperglycemia in the postabsorptive state.[58] Moreover, glucagon is inappropriately released in response to a meal and may be responsible in part for postprandial excursions seen in T2DM.[58]

SUMMARY

The pathophysiology of T2DM is characterized by interrelated deficits observed in the liver, muscle, brain, adipose tissue, kidneys, GI tract, and pancreas. Insulin resistance and β cell dysfunction progress along a spectrum of disease from hyperinsulinemia to impaired glucose tolerance, hyperglycemia, and frank insulin deficiency. Understanding the relationships between these multiple pathways will help clinicians target treatment using different approaches that are sensitive to each patient's unique presentation. Early and intensive interventions improve outcomes and limit long-term complications.

DISCLOSURE

The authors have nothing to disclose.

REFERENCES

1. Defronzo RA. Banting lecture: from the triumvirate to the ominous octet: a new paradigm for the treatment of type 2 diabetes mellitus. Diabetes 2009;58(4):773–95.

2. Defronzo RA. Lilly lecture 1987: the triumvirate: beta-cell, muscle, liver. A collusion responsible for NIDDM. Diabetes 1988;37(6):667–87.

3. American Diabetes Association. Standards of medical care in diabetes—2019. Diabetes Care 2019;42(1):S1–193.

4. Kautzky-Willer A, Harreiter J, Pacini G. Sex and gender differences in risk, pathophysiology and complications of type 2 diabetes mellitus. Endocr Rev 2016; 34(3):278–316.

5. White MG, Shaw JAM, Taylor R. Type 2 diabetes: the pathologic basis of reversible B-Cell dysfunction. Diabetes Care 2016;(39):2080–8.

6. Jager S, Wahl S, Kroger J, et al. Genetic variants including markers from the exome chip and metabolite traits of type 2 diabetes. Sci Rep 2017;7(1):6037.

7. Thomas MC. Glycemic exposure, glycemic control and metabolic karma in diabetic complications. Adv Chronic Kidney Dis 2014;21(3):311–7.

8. Berezin A. Metabolic memory phenomenon in diabetes mellitus: achieving and perspectives. Diabetes Metab Syndr 2016;10(2 Suppl 1):S176–83.

9. Vargas E, Carrillo Sepulveda MA. Biochemistry, insulin metabolic effects. Last update: April 21, 2019. StatPearls [Internet]. Available at: https://www.ncbi.nlm.nih.gov/books/NBK525983/. Accessed June 30, 2019.

10. Petersen MC, Shulman GI. Mechanisms of insulin action and insulin resistance. Physiol Rev 2018;98:2133–223.

11. Lundquist MH, Almby K, Abrahamsson, et al. Is the brain a key player in glucose regulation and development of type 2 diabetes? Front Physiol 2019;10:457.

12. Kahn CR, Crettaz M. Insulin receptors and the molecular mechanism of insulin action. Diabetes Metab Rev 1985;1(1–2):5–32.

13. Sattar N, Gill JMR. Type 2 diabetes as a disease of ectopic fat? BMC Med 2014;12:123.

14. Barbarroja N, Lopez-Pedrera C, Garrido-Sanchez L, et al. Progression from high insulin resistance to type 2 diabetes does not entail additional visceral adipose tissue inflammation. PLoS One 2012;7(10):e48155.

15. Petersen MC, Vatner DF, Shulman GI. Regulation of hepatic glucose metabolism in health and disease. Nat Rev Endocrinol 2017;13(10):572–87.

16. Haeusler RA, Hartil K, Bhavapriya V, et al. Integrated control of hepatic lipogenesis vs. glucose production requires FoxO transcription factors. Nat Commun 2015;5:5190.

17. Pajvani UB, Accili D. The new biology of diabetes. Diabetologia 2015;58(11):2459–68.

18. Bonnadonna RC, Del Prato S, Bonora E, et al. Roles of glucose transport and glucose phosphorylation in muscle insulin resistance of NIDDM. Diabetes 1996;45:915–25.

19. Liu J, Liu Z. Muscle insulin resistance and the inflamed microvasculature: fire from within. Int J Mol Sci 2019;20(3) [pii:E562].

20. Lee Y, Chakraborty S, Meininger CJ, et al. Insulin resistance disrupts cell integrity, mitochondrial function and inflammatory signaling in lymphatic endothelium. Microcirculation 2018;25:e12492.

21. Shoelson SE, Lee J, Goldfine AB. Inflammation and insulin resistance. J Clin Invest 2006;116(7):1793–801.

22. Inoue H, Ogawa W, Asakawa A, et al. Role of hepatic STAT3 in brain-insulin action on hepatic glucose production. Cell Metab 2006;(3):267–75.

23. Koch L, Wunderlich T, Seibler J, et al. Central insulin action regulates peripheral glucose and fat metabolism in mice. J Clin Invest 2008;118:2132–47.

24. Kishore P, Boucai L, Zhang K, et al. Activation of KATP channels suppresses glucose production in humans. Diabetes 2016;65(9):2569–79.

25. Filippi BM, Bassiri A, Abraham MA, et al. Insulin signals through the dorsal vagal complex to regulate energy balance. Diabetes 2014;63:892–9.

26. Abraham MA, Filippi BM, Kang GM, et al. Insulin action in the hypothalamus and dorsal vagal complex. Exp Physiol 2014;99:1104–9.

27. Kern W, Benedict C, Schultes B, et al. Low cerebrospinal fluid insulin levels in obese humans. Diabetologia 2006;49(11):2790–2.
28. Del Prado S. Role of glucotoxicity and lipotoxicity in the pathophysiology of type 2 diabetes mellitus and emerging treatment strategies. Diabetic Med 2009;26: 1185–92.
29. Bodis K, Roden M. Energy metabolism of white adipose tissue and insulin resistance in humans. Eur J Clin Invest 2018;48:e13017.
30. Xie X, Zhengping Y, Sinha S, et al. Proteomics analyses of subcutaneous adipocytes reveal novel abnormalities in human insulin resistance. Obesity (Silver Spring) 2016;24(7):1506–14.
31. Burhans MS, Hagman DK, Kuzma JN, et al. Contribution of adipose tissue inflammation to the development of type 2 diabetes. Compr Physiol 2019;9(1):1–58.
32. Wang ZV, Scherer PE. Adiponectin, the past two decades. J Mol Cell Biol 2016; 8(2):93–100.
33. Akbari M, Hassan-Zadeh V. IL-6 signalling pathways and the development of type 2 diabetes. Inflammopharmacology 2018;(26):685–98.
34. Gerich JE. Role of the kidney in normal glucose homeostasis and in the hyperglycaemia of diabetes mellitus: therapeutic implications. Diabet Med 2010;27: 136–42.
35. Costanzo LS. Renal physiology. Physiology. 6th edition. Philadelphia: Elsevier; 2018. p. 245–310.
36. Meyer C, Woerle HJ, Dostou JM, et al. Abnormal renal, hepatic, and muscle glucose metabolism following glucose ingestion in type 2 diabetes. Am J Physiol Endocrinol Metab 2004;287:E1049–56.
37. Farber SJ, Berger EY, Earle DP. Effect of diabetes and insulin on the maximum capacity of the renal tubules to reabsorb glucose. J Clin Invest 1951;30(2): 125–9.
38. Vallon V, Thomson SC. Targeting renal glucose reabsorption to treat hyperglycaemia: the pleiotropic effects of SGLT2 inhibition. Diabetologia 2017;60(2): 215–25.
39. Wanner C, Lachin JM, Inzucchi SE, et al. Empagliflozin and clinical outcomes in patients with type 2 diabetes mellitus, established cardiovascular disease and chronic kidney disease. Circulation 2018;137:119–29.
40. Nauck MA, Meier JJ. Incretin hormones: their role in health and disease. Diabetes Obes Metab 2018;20(Suppl. 1):5–21.
41. Nauck MA, Meier JJ. The incretin effect in healthy individuals and those with type 2 diabetes: physiology, pathophysiology, and response to therapeutic interventions. Lancet Diabetes Endocrinol 2016;(4):525–36.
42. Yang M, Wang J, Wu S, et al. Duodenal GLP-1 signaling regulates hepatic glucose production through a PKC-d-dependent neurocircuitry. Cell Death Dis 2017;8(2):e2609.
43. Calanna S, Christensen M, Holst JJ, et al. Secretion of glucagon-like peptide-1 in patients with type 2 diabetes mellitus: systematic review and meta-analyses of clinical studies. Diabetologia 2013;56(5):965–72.
44. Lim GE, Huang GJ, Flora N, et al. Insulin regulates glucagon-like peptide-1 secretion from the enteroendocrine L cell. Endocrinology 2009;150(2):580–91.
45. Hinnen D. Glucagon-like peptide 1 receptor agonists for type 2 diabetes. Diabetes Spectr 2017;30(3):202–10.
46. Bethel MA, Patel RA, Merrill P, et al. Cardiovascular outcomes with glucagon-like peptide-1 receptor agonists in patients with type 2 diabetes: a meta-analysis. Lancet Diabetes Endocrinol 2018;6(2):105–13.

47. Deacon CF. Physiology and pharmacology of DPP-4 in glucose homeostasis and the treatment of type 2 diabetes. Front Endocrinol (Lausanne) 2019;10:80.
48. Saisho Y. Pancreas volume and fat deposition in diabetes and normal physiology: consideration of the interplay between endocrine and exocrine pancreas. Rev Diabet Stud 2016;13(2–3):132–47.
49. Costanzo LS. Chapter 8: Gastrointestinal physiology. In: Physiology, sixth edition, pp. 339–93.
50. Oakie A, Wang R. B-cell receptor tyrosine kinases in controlling insulin secretion and exocytotic machinery; c-Kit and insulin receptor. Endocrinology 2018;159:3813–21.
51. Bi P, Kuang S. Notch signaling as a novel regulator of metabolism. Trends Endocrinol Metab 2015;26(5):248–55.
52. Butler AE, Robertson RP, Hernandez R, et al. Beta cell nuclear musculoaponeurotic fibrosarcoma oncogene family A (MafA) is deficient in type 2 diabetes. Diabetologia 2012;55(11):2985–8.
53. Iype T, Taylor GD, Ziesmann SM, et al. The transcriptional repressor NKx6.1 also functions as a deoxyribonucleic acid context-dependent transcriptional activator during pancreatic B-cell differentiation; evidence for feedback activation of the nkx6.1 gene by Nkx6.1. Mol Endocrinol 2004;18(6):1363–75.
54. Fujimoto K, Polonsky KS. Pdx 1 and other factors that regulate pancreatic B-cell survival. Diabetes Obes Metab 2009;11(Suppl 4):30–7.
55. Bartolome A, Zhu C, Sussel L, et al. Notch signaling dynamically regulates adult B cell proliferation and maturity. J Clin Invest 2019;129(1):268–80.
56. Hogan MF, Hull RL. The islet endothelial cell: a novel contributor to beta cell secretory dysfunction in diabetes. Diabetologia 2017;60(6):952–9.
57. Lund A. On the role of the gut in diabetic hyperglucagonaemia. Dan Med J 2017; 64(4) [pii:B5340]. Available at: https://ugeskriftet.dk/dmj/role-gut-diabetic-hyperglucagonaemia.
58. Girard J. Glucagon, a key factor in the pathophysiology of type 2 diabetes. Biochimie 2017;143:33–6.
59. Reaven GM, Chen YDI, Golay A, et al. Documentation of hyperglucagonemia throughout the day in nonobese and obese patients with noninsulin dependent diabetes mellitus. J Clin Endocrinol Metab 1987;64(1):106–10.

Putting the Patient in Charge

Melissa Rodzen, MMS, PA-C[a,b,c,*]

KEYWORDS

- Diabetes management • Patient-centered care • Glycemic control
- Lifestyle modification • Diabetic treatment compliance
- Barriers to diabetes treatment • Patient empowerment • Diabetes self-care

KEY POINTS

- The patient-centered care model is the cornerstone of diabetes management and leads to improved patient care.
- Patients who feel empowered and involved in their care are more likely to improve self-care measures.
- When goals are clear, specific, and individualized, barriers are acknowledged and lifestyle changes are more readily accepted.

INTRODUCTION

The days of medical paternalism are gone and the days of advising lifestyle changes in the form of "lose weight and increase physical activity" are numbered. As time goes on, the importance of discarding standardized advice in favor of individualized, patient-centered care is becoming the cornerstone of diabetes management. The American Diabetes Association (ADA) recommends a "patient-centered communication style" but offers little guidance for practitioners about how to involve patients. References to patient self-management and education programs are frequently mentioned in diabetes literature as effective methods for lifestyle modification but are infrequently explained, defined, or discussed as a standard for practice.[1]

Diabetes is a complex, multifactorial disease that permeates every aspect of a patient's life and often the lives of their friends and families. Implementing a patient-centered care model to provide individualized care extends past the A1C

---

[a] American Academy of Physician Assistants, Alexandria, VA, USA; [b] American Association of Clinical Endocrinologists, Jacksonville, FL, USA; [c] American Diabetes Association, Arlington, VA, USA
* Middle Country Endocrinology, 285 Middle Country Road, Suite 105, Smithtown, NY 11787.
E-mail address: melissa.rodzen@gmail.com

Physician Assist Clin 5 (2020) 135–142
https://doi.org/10.1016/j.cpha.2019.11.003
2405-7991/20/© 2019 Elsevier Inc. All rights reserved.

to improving not only physical health but also emotional, mental, social, and financial well-being. It is a model that addresses not only the goals of health care providers but also the needs of the patient.[2] Acknowledging that these 2 sets of goals are often not aligned is imperative when identifying barriers to effective diabetes care.

Although it is true that both providers and patients report controlling glucose levels among the highest goals in diabetes management, studies comparing strategies for obtaining this goal are often discordant. For example, providers are more likely to perceive additional measures such as blood pressure control, cholesterol control, and following reduced calorie diets as the most important measures of diabetes care. Patients, however, were more likely to report avoiding insulin, coming off medications, and decreasing physical discomforts of treatment as primary goals. Similarly, perceived barriers to care were often very different as defined by patients and providers.[3]

When creating a patient-centered plan for diabetes management, the first step should always be a goal-directed discussion between the provider and the patient to identify both goals and personal barriers to achieving positive outcomes.

THE MOTIVATIONAL INTERVIEW: ESTABLISHING GOALS

When discussing goals and barriers to care, there are several techniques for eliciting important information from patients. Motivational interviewing is a useful tool that is implemented in a variety of specialties from smoking cessation to eating disorder management, which all require behavioral modification. Although many providers report feeling confident about sharing educational information with patients and discussing treatment options through directive approaches, they often feel much less able to help patients implement lifestyle changes to reach their goals. In fact, nearly 40% of practitioners felt unable to influence improvements in diet or exercise habits in their patients.[4] The motivational interview not only helps the provider and patient begin communication but also involves the patient and encourages active discussion about risks, benefits, problematic behaviors, and readiness for change.[5]

The motivational interview was initially developed in 1983 in addiction medicine as a more goal-directed style of communication with which to work in collaboration with patients. It uses social learning theory to not only guide the patient to recognize target behaviors in need of change but also to build self-confidence and empowerment to change their own lives and behaviors. This style of interview is intended to discuss with a patient their specific situation and motivation for or against behavior modification using a series of steps[5] (**Box 1**).

Box 1
The motivational interview

Steps
1. Engaging with the patient to address fears, goals, and possible barriers to care.
2. The most attention should be placed on the patient's most desired goal, which involves behavior they are most ready to change.
3. Empowering the patient with the sense that they have the ability to change.
4. Setting specific goals and helping the patient develop a detailed plan to reach those goals.

Data from Rippe JM. Lifestyle Medicine. Boca Raton: Taylor & Francis; 2019.

COMMUNICATION STRATEGIES

When conducting the patient-centered interview, it is important to keep several communication strategies in mind. Although there are few studies evaluating the effectiveness of A1C reduction as a result of the motivational interview, the psychological impacts are well documented.

Traditionally, medicine uses the frequent use of closed questioning. This impersonal interview is designed for data collection, but when treating the patient with diabetes, research shows patients improve when they are engaged in their care. They are more likely to offer more information from their own frame of reference (rather than the provider's) when answering open-ended questions.[5]

IDENTIFYING BARRIERS

A barrier may be any rationalization preventing a desired course of action: financial concerns, emotional or physical discomfort, social pressures, inconvenience, or any perception that a given cost is greater than the proposed benefit. Awareness of barriers and contributing factors (race, gender, education, health literacy, socioeconomic status, mental health) are essential to identifying any particular individual's reasons for nonadherence. This requires self-awareness from the patient perspective and understanding from the provider perspective.[4]

Many studies have evaluated reported and perceived barriers to achieving goals in diabetes care from the patient and provider point of reference. These studies span a variety of socioeconomic, ethnic, and environmental backgrounds. Awareness of barriers to care as well as motivational barriers is important to identify during the patient interview, as they often influence patient and provider behavior and success.[5] It is not surprising that the most frequent difficulty reported by patients with diabetes is adherence to diet and exercise regimens.[4] However, the reasons for nonadherence can be as diverse as the diabetic population itself, with each individual reporting numerous influences on their behaviors. Furthermore, one must also consider barriers from the provider's perspective preventing successful patient guidance when investigating and creating treatment plans to overcome these barriers.

PATIENT BARRIERS

When designing a patient-centered approach to care, more attention is given to a patient's mental health, health literacy, abilities, resources, and opinions than in traditional medicine. Research has demonstrated on multiple accounts that psychological barriers are strongly related to A1C control and an individual's overall sense of well-being.[3,6,7] Patients with Hgb A1C greater than 10% report higher rates of depression, lack of confidence, and overall lack of social support regarding their management compared with their peers with lower A1C levels.[8]

Socioeconomic status also plays a strong role in long-term management of diabetes. Patients from a lower socioeconomic status are more likely to miss appointments, lack education to understand diabetes laboratory discussions and implications of poor control, have elevated A1C values, suffer from depression, miss preventative care services, are unable to afford medications, and are less likely to receive specialized care.[8]

Understanding the reasons behind a patient's nonadherence or difficulty achieving effective diabetes self-management behavior is essential for overcoming obstacles in diabetes treatment. The list of barriers is infinite. It is important to demonstrate interest in uncovering patient's barriers to achieve A1C reduction and a sense of well-being.

PROVIDER BARRIERS

Overall, providers are more likely to report logistics around diabetes management as barriers. These 5 items are cited by providers as barriers to better outcomes: limited time, unclear guidelines, lack of health care system support, difficulty motivating patients, and issues with health literacy.[3] The list of possible barriers from a provider's perspective is just as numerous as possible patient barriers and may vary from patient to patient for the same provider. It is important for providers to be mindful of their own barriers to providing care and to work with patients to overcome them. At times, this will mean abandoning standardized approaches to therapy in favor of individualized approaches to improve care.[9,10]

OVERCOMING BARRIERS AND IMPLEMENTING CHANGE

Patient empowerment is the cornerstone of patient-centered care and effective self-management. Often, when patients believe that they are able to influence the negative impact of their disease, they are more likely to share their goals with their providers.[3] When patients report higher levels of diabetes education, they are more likely to share similar goals as their providers and are more likely to report improved confidence as well as understanding of self-care behaviors.[3,6] When creating a care plan, it is important to use the motivational interview to evaluate perceived barriers by the patients and readiness for change to build rapport and a sense of empowerment. Research suggests that patients who believe they can overcome barriers are more likely to do so. This accentuates the importance of identifying specific goals, barriers to goals, and plans that are tailored to each individual patient's wants and needs.

THE IMPORTANCE OF SPECIFICITY

A patient-centered approach must consider each individual's concerns, limitations, and motivations for change in order to be effective while keeping in mind the potential differences between provider and patient perspectives. This is especially important when attempting to help patients overcome barriers to lifestyle modification.

For example, when comparing responses from both diabetes educators and patients, educators rated measures of judgment and self-control as more prominent barriers. Patients, on the other hand, tended to rate physical limitations higher. Nearly one-third of patients reported physical limitations were "most or all" or "usually or always" barriers to completing exercise plans, whereas educators only estimated physical limitations as a barrier 6% of the time. Diabetes educators reported portion sizes, adhering to diet plans while eating out, and snack temptations as higher barriers than patients. Patients were more concerned that meal plans did not contain their favorite foods.[4] This demonstrates differences in assumed barriers, goals, and likely perceptions regarding appropriate diet or exercise options.

NUTRITION, EXERCISE, AND WEIGHT LOSS

Specific instructions regarding nutritional management are essential when setting goals with patients. Many people have misconceptions when it comes to nutritional needs, yet advice from providers is often vague. There are numerous studies detailing consistent results showing A1C reduction with specific nutritional advice.[11] Nutritional recommendations should be personalized per patient and are best delivered by a registered dietician familiar with medical nutritional therapy.[11–13] **Box 2** offers suggestions and guidance for specific topics of discussion for evidence-based nutritional strategies associated with weight loss and A1C reduction.

Exercise also plays a major role in maintaining a healthy lifestyle but is often difficult for patients to accomplish for a variety of reasons. As a component of the motivational interview, benefits of exercise should be discussed with the patient in relation to specific goals and concerns while being mindful of potential barriers. In addition to weight loss, improvements in aerobic fitness translate to increased insulin sensitivity and improved glucose levels. When creating specific goals with patients, one should define meaningful exercise and encourage gradual increases in activity. Initial goals should be achievable at patient's current ability and gradually increased. A generalized example of recommendations and effects of exercise can be found in **Tables 1–3**.

MAKING THE CHANGE

Research shows that the provider-patient relationships have significant impact on patient outcomes. When providers are engaged in patient-centered care, patient self-management, adherence to treatment plans, and overall satisfaction is improved.[14] Improvements in patient motivation, mental health, and application of education have demonstrated measurable improvements in A1C and overall patient satisfaction. Using the patient-centered approach to improve care, providers have an opportunity to positively affect coping skills, mental health, and overall well-being of our patients.[14,17]

Box 2
Examples of specific nutritional talking points

- Referring for additional nutritional counseling
  - Patients should be referred to a registered dietician at diagnosis to establish structured medical nutritional therapy.
  - Research demonstrates medical nutritional counseling to significantly lower Hgb A1C in type 1 and type 2 diabetic patients.
  - ADA recommends 3 to 4 encounters within 6 months with a registered dietician lasting 45 minutes to 90 minutes followed by at least yearly follow-up.
  - Improved results when combined with cognitive behavioral therapy.

- For patients on insulin
  - Focused carb counting, meal planning, and appropriate insulin dosing

- Specific weight loss targets
  - Establishing specific weight loss goal—ADA recommends 7% to 8.5% initial body weight with realistic milestone targets
  - Five hundred calorie deficit per day is expected to yield about 1lb per week weight loss
  - Discussing caloric needs based on height and energy expenditure to plan realistic expectations and expected rate of weight loss based on caloric intake
  - Weekly self-weighing to prevent discouragement from daily fluctuations

- Consider barriers to adequate nutrition
  - Access to grocery stores
  - Ability to prepare food
  - Personal tastes
  - Comorbidities influencing diet
  - Depression or lack of social support

Data from Warshaw H, Daly A, Franz M, Kulkarni K. The Evidence for the Effectiveness of Medical Nutrition Therapy in Diabetes Management. Diabetes Care. Evert AB, Boucher JL, Cypress M, et al. Nutrition Therapy Recommendations for the Management of Adults With Diabetes. Diabetes Care.

Table 1
Communication strategies

Do...	Avoid...

• Use open-ended questions
  ○ "What do you think about the new medication we started last month?"
  ○ "How do you feel when you try to exercise?"
  ○ "What part of managing your glucose levels do you find the most difficult?"
	• Closed "yes" or "no" questions
	  ○ "Are you checking your glucose levels 4 times per day?"
	  ○ "You're not having any hypoglycemia, are you?"
	  ○ "Do you feel like you are exercising enough?"

• Provide positive comments regarding patient's motivations, intentions, and efforts
  ○ "You keep very organized records of your glucose levels. This is very helpful for us to target why you are having lows."
  ○ "I can really see the positive changes you've made in your diet. With a few more changes we can discuss discontinuing some of your medications."
  ○ "It isn't easy to find time to exercise, but you've increased from one or twice per month to once per week! Your hard work is making a difference."
	• Focusing solely on quantitative change without acknowledging effort
	  ○ "Your blood pressure has improved, but your cholesterol levels are still too high. Eat fewer saturated fats."
	  ○ "It looks like the medication change we made during last visit is working—your Hgb A1C is improved."
	  ○ "You should be exercising 3 times per week."

• Participate with active listening
  ○ Maintain eye contact while conversing with a patient
  ○ Observe nonverbal behaviors
  ○ Acknowledge patient concerns before responding with your opinion
  ○ Let patients finish speaking before responding
  ○ Provide a brief summary of patient statements to show understanding and attention
	• Passive or reactive listening
	  ○ Write prescription refills while your patient talks
	  ○ Dismiss nonverbal cues
	  ○ Disagree with patient statement before acknowledging concern/comment
	  ○ Interrupt
	  ○ Wait for the patient to finish speaking and then move on

• Provide advice and information
  ○ "I know you have been working hard to control your glucose levels and lose weight. There is one medication that may help you reach those goals. I'll tell you about the risks and benefits and you can ask me any questions and tell me if you think it is something you would like to try."
  ○ "You have mentioned you want to decrease the number of medications you're taking. Here are possible alternatives and the risks of stopping. What are your thoughts?"
	• Making decisions for patients
	  ○ "I'm starting you on this medication to lower your glucose levels."
	  ○ "You have mentioned that decreasing the number of medications you're taking is a priority for you, but you are stable on them so we won't make any changes at this time."

Data from Rippe JM. Lifestyle Medicine. Boca Raton: Taylor & Francis; 2019.

Table 2
Reported barriers to care

Reported by Patients	Reported by Providers

• Socioeconomic Barriers
  ○ More likely to forego treatment due to cost concerns
  ○ Less likely to have regular follow-up
  ○ Less likely to receive specialist care
	• Time Burden
	  ○ Limited resources to address all aspects of diabetic care during visits
	  ○ Frequently changing medications and guidelines making current recommendations unclear

• Physical and Psychological Barriers
  ○ Lack of confidence regarding ability to influence disease control or progression
  ○ Lack of social support
  ○ Lack of systemic support
  ○ Difficulty initiating behavioral modification
  ○ Comorbidities or depression
  ○ Physical limitations or pain preventing patient from following recommendations
	• Medications
	  ○ Numerous medications with varying responses from patients
	  ○ Multiple medications often needed to control glucose levels
	  ○ Frequent medication adjustments necessary
	  ○ Encouraging patient compliance with medication
	  ○ Treatments sometimes cause more symptoms than the disease

• Educational/Health Care Literacy
  ○ Difficulty using equipment to test glucose levels
  ○ Lack of understanding of laboratory results and implications of poor control
  ○ Limited time with providers to discuss disease process, complications, treatment plans, and the importance of control
	• Patient Education
	  ○ Patients are sometimes resistant to treat hyperglycemia due to lack of symptoms
	  ○ Provider and patient goals or priorities misaligned
	  ○ Cultural or language differences limiting education and communication effectiveness
	  ○ Providers are unable to directly change patient diet or lifestyle

Data from Refs.[3,4,8]

Table 3
Examples of specific exercise recommendations

• Aerobic exercise	• Suggested starting program 10 min per day with gradual increases in duration and intensity • Eventual target of 30–45 min exercise with target heart rate 50%–70% maximum at least 3 d per week • 60–75 min of walking or 35 min of jogging daily to achieve weight loss
• Resistance training	• 3 sessions of weight training at 60% maximum heart rate from 20 min to 30 min per session over 10 wk • 3 sets of 8–10 repetitions per weight group • May be ideal for patients with mobility limitations • Yields significant reduction of plasma glucose levels and Hgb A1C reduction

Data from Klein, Samuel, Sheard, et al. Weight management through lifestyle modification for the prevention and management of type 2 diabetes: rationale and strategies. A statement of the American Diabetes Association, the North American Association for the Study of Obesity, and the American Society for Clinical Nutrition. OUP Academic. Bweir1 S, Al-Jarrah2 M, Almalty1 A-M, Smirnova3 IV, Lesya, Stehno-Bittel3 L. Resistance exercise training lowers HbA1c more than aerobic training in adults with type 2 diabetes. Diabetology & Metabolic Syndrome.

DISCLOSURE

None.

REFERENCES

1. American Diabetes Association. Standards of medical care in diabetes-2019 abridged for primary care providers. Clin Diabetes 2019;37(1):11–34.
2. Das LT, Abramson EL, Kaushal R. High-need, high-cost patients offer solutions for improving their care and reducing costs. NEJM Catal 2019;2019. pii: https://catalyst.nejm.org/high-need-high-cost-patients-solutions/.
3. Heisler M, Vijan S, Anderson RM, et al. When do patients and their physicians agree on diabetes treatment goals and strategies, and what difference does it make? J Gen Intern Med 2003;18(11):893–902.
4. Pun SPY, Coates V, Phil D, et al. Barriers to the self-care of type 2 diabetes from both patients' and providers' perspectives: literature review. J Nurs Healthc Chr III 2009. Available at: https://onlinelibrary.wiley.com/doi/full/10.1111/j.1365-2702.2008.01000.x.
5. Rippe JM. Are we ready to practice lifestyle medicine? Am J Med 2019;132(1):6–8.
6. Heisler M, Bouknight RR, Hayward RA, et al. The relative importance of physician communication, participatory decision making, and patient understanding in diabetes self-management. J Gen Intern Med 2002;17(4):243–52.
7. Dogru A, Ovayolu N, Ovayolu O. The effect of motivational interview persons with diabetes on self-management and metabolic variables. J Pak Med Assoc 2019;69(3):294–300.
8. Mcbrien KA, Naugler C, Ivers N, et al. Barriers to care in patients with diabetes and poor glycemic control—A cross-sectional survey. PLoS One 2017;12(5):e0176135.
9. Subramanian S, Hirsch IB. Personalized diabetes management: moving from algorithmic to individualized therapy. Diabetes Spectr 2014;27(2):87–91.
10. Pastors JG, Warshaw H, Daly A, et al. The evidence for the effectiveness of medical nutrition therapy in diabetes management. Diabetes Care 2002;25(3):608–13.
11. Evert AB, Boucher JL, Cypress M, et al. Nutrition therapy recommendations for the management of adults with diabetes. Diabetes Care 2013;36(11):3821–42.
12. Klein S, Sheard NF, Pi-Sunyer X, et al. Weight management through lifestyle modification for the prevention and management of type 2 diabetes: rationale and strategies: a statement of the American Diabetes Association, the North American Association for the Study of Obesity, and the American Society for Clinical Nutrition. Diabetes Care 2004;27(8):2067–73.
13. Freeman-Hildreth Y, Aron D, Cola PA, et al. Coping with diabetes: provider attributes that influence type 2 diabetes adherence. PLoS One 2019;14(4):e0214713.
14. Norris SL, Engelgau MM, Narayan KMV. Effectiveness of self-management training in type 2 diabetes. Diabetes Care 2001;24(3):561–87.

The Diabetic Grocery Cart
Evidence-Based Nutrition Recommendations for the Practitioner

Ciara Mitchell, MA, RD

KEYWORDS

- Diabetic diet • Patient-centered care • Diabetic education

KEY POINTS

- A challenging aspect of diabetes care to understand for the practitioner and the patient is diet.
- Many practitioners lack knowledge and confidence when managing a patient's diet.
- Practical dietary advice is important for dietary patients.

INTRODUCTION

Diabetes is a growing epidemic in the United States. In 2017, more than 30 million adults had diabetes and these numbers are expected to triple by 2050.[1,2] Diabetes is ranked as the seventh leading cause of death in the United States and is the number 1 cause of kidney failure, blindness, and lower limb amputation.[2] In 2014, more than 7 million US hospital discharges were reported as diabetes related.[3]

Those with diabetes are at an increased risk for microvascular and macrovascular comorbidities, including hypertension, stroke, cardiovascular disease (CVD), retinopathy, neuropathy, and nephropathy.[4] Premature mortality, morbidity and the relative risk for death owing to CVD are 3-fold higher in persons with diabetes compared with the general population.[5]

Among the most prevalent risk factors for development of diabetes is obesity and lack of physical activity.[6,7] These are both modifiable risk factors and early intervention can help to delay or prevent complications. Dietary management is vital in prevention, control, and managing of diabetes, but many do not have access to a dietician. Although there are many risk factors for developing type 2 diabetes mellitus (T2DM), obesity plays the greatest role. More than 60% of people with T2DM are obese (body mass index $\geq$30 kg/m^2).[7] Although rates of T2DM are higher in older populations, with the growing epidemic of childhood obesity, rates are increasing in children and adolescents.[5,7] Treatment recommendations are often focused on

University of Alabama at Birmingham, Richard Arrington Blvd S, Birmingham, AL 35233, USA
E-mail address: Ciaramitchell@uabmc.edu

Physician Assist Clin 5 (2020) 143–152
https://doi.org/10.1016/j.cpha.2019.11.004
2405-7991/20/© 2019 Elsevier Inc. All rights reserved.

physicianassistant.theclinics.com

achieving weight loss among those who are overweight through diet and lifestyle modification.[7,8]

THE DIABETIC DIET COMES OF AGE

Historically, diabetes was viewed as a death sentence by both physicians and patients. Those with diabetes died shortly after being diagnosed.[9] In the early 1900s, before insulin was discovered, physicians recommended very low-carbohydrate (carb) diets with the omission of sugar. Some physicians even recommended diets just short of starvation.[9] Even though patients following these diets would extend their lives by an extra 1 or 2 years, many of them suffered from a poor quality of life.[9] In the 1920s, the perspective of diabetes management changed drastically when Dr Frederick Banting and his team in Toronto, Ontario, Canada, discovered insulin.[10] In 1922, he and his colleagues tested insulin on the first human subject, a 14-year-old boy named Leonard Thompson. This was successful and Thompson lived 14 more years, eventually succumbing to pneumonia and not his diabetes.[11]

With the introduction of insulin, less restricted diets were prescribed. In the mid-1930s, after the discovery of insulin, high-carb diets (66% carbs) were recommended. This was owing to the severe hypoglycemia often associated with insulin. Studies during this time showed that high-carb diets were improving glucose tolerance and preventing decreases in glucose levels.[9]

In the 1940s, unrestricted diets were recommended and well-accepted among the diabetic population. In the 1950s, it was noted that those with diabetes were dying at a high rate from vascular disease. This signaled an end to the unrestricted diet era.[9] In the late 1950s, representatives from the American Diabetes Association (ADA) recommended lower carb diets (about 40% of total calories), avoidance of refined sugars, and moderate fat intake with emphasis on low-fat or unsaturated fat products for the dietary treatment of diabetes.[10] This became known as the ADA diabetic diet and the first of many ADA recommendations.[12]

DIABETES MANAGEMENT GOALS

Patients with diabetes cannot effectively break down carbs into energy sources; therefore, diet therapy plays a crucial role in meeting diabetes management goals. Thus, the ADA has developed a set of nutrition related goals for optimal diabetes control.[13] These goals include achieving a glycated hemoglobin (HbA1c) of 7% or less, maintaining a blood pressure of less than 140/80 mm Hg, achieving a low-density lipoprotein of 100 mg/dL or less, a triglyceride level of less than 150 mg/dL, and high-density lipoprotein of greater than 40 mg/dL for men and greater than 50 mg/dL for women, and achieving healthy body weight.[14]

Effectively managing diabetes requires blood sugar control.[15] The Joslin Diabetes Center recommends people with diabetes aim for a fasting blood sugar of 70 to 130 mg/dL, a postprandial blood sugar less than 180 mg/dL, and a bedtime blood sugar of 90 to 150 mg/dL.[15]

Although achieving diabetes management goals are a top priority, doing so can be difficult owing to the multicomplex nature and disease progression of diabetes. Effective nutrition education can prevent complications for many, but the abundance of information in the media, online, and in news articles, can lead to confusion for all concerned.

Although evidence shows the delivery of nutrition education is best done by a registered dietitian or certified diabetes educator, it is recognized that registered dietitians and certified diabetes educators are not always available given the growing number of patients with diabetes.[16] Thus, nutrition and diabetes education is often delivered by other providers who are well-trained in diabetic management but have limited formal nutrition training, have low confidence in discussing dietary matters, and lack knowledge in dietary counseling and recommendations.[17]

To successfully manage a patient with diabetes, one must know the current nutritional recommendations, the myths circulating on social media and the Internet, and appreciate the importance of shared decision making.

CONFLICTING DIET MESSAGES

There is a common consensus that healthy eating patterns play a key role in managing diabetes. However, for many with diabetes, determining what is healthy eating is a challenge. Today, with a plethora of dietary information and conflicting diet messages from the media, family members, and peers. Adding to the confusion and frustration are dietary instructions from health care providers, which may be contradictory. For example, some are told, "eat more protein and avoid the carbs," some told, "avoid sugar and limit your carbs," and some are told, "just eat everything in moderation." These diet messages are hard to follow, leading to the labeling of patients as nonadherent. Advertisements have become the snake oil salesman of the 21st century offering wonder treatments, cures in a bottle, and miraculous weight loss with little effort by the patient.

To help clarify and accurately educate patients on dietary recommendations, the ADA developed a grading system to categorize the evidence that makes up the basis for nutrition recommendations.[14] This grading system is based on findings from randomized controlled trials, meta-analyses, and Cochrane reviews. This information enables practitioners without formal nutrition training to deliver evidenced-based dietary advice to patients with diabetes.

NO MORE ONE-SIZE-FITS-ALL APPROACH

With emerging evidence, a more comprehensive approach to diabetes management is recommended. The ADA recognizes there is not a one-size-fits-all approach to nutrition in diabetes. Instead of encouraging 1 diet such as the ADA's diabetic diet, as previously recommended, the goal of nutrition therapy is an individualized approach. Goals should be based on the patient's personal and cultural preferences, while maintaining pleasurable eating by providing positive messages around food choices. Instead of focusing on single foods or macronutrients and micronutrients, the patient should be provided with practical tools for day-to-day meal planning. There are a number of evidenced-based nutrition strategies that providers can use and incorporate into their interactions when working with their patients with diabetes.

Address and Encourage Weight Loss

For overweight or obese adults with T2DM, decreasing caloric intake while maintaining a healthful eating pattern can promote weight loss and improve clinical outcomes. A modest weight loss (eg, $\geq$5%) may improve blood sugars, blood pressure, and lipids; this is strategy especially effective in the early stages of the disease process. Achieving modest weight loss requires lifestyle interventions such as nutrition counseling, increased physical activity, and behavior changes. Preventing weight gain is equally important as losing weight.[14]

STRATEGIES TO CONSIDER
Conduct Lifestyle Counseling

Lifestyle counseling focuses on behaviors rather than providing diet advice or information. For example, consider the patient who has gained significant weight since the last visit and whose HbA1c is greater than 8.5%. You are concerned about the weight gain and blood sugar control. Rather than saying, "You need to lose weight and get your blood sugars under control," ask a series of open-ended questions such as, "Tell me a little bit about what you eat," and "I noticed you've gained weight since your last appointment; what do you think has changed?" During this brief counseling session, you discover that the patient snacks from the vending machine 5 to 6 times a day because of work stress. You and the patient both discuss strategies or healthy behaviors to adopt when under stress. Together, you decide it is best to go on a short walk at work to relieve stress and encourage the patient to bring healthy snacks rather than relying on the vending machine.

Focus on Calorie Reduction and Increasing Physical Activity

Rather than advising patients to avoid single foods or macronutrients or adopting certain diets, encourage and discuss ways to reduce total caloric intake. Those who eat more calories than they burn gain weight; therefore, patients with diabetes should focus on consuming fewer and burning more calories to promote weight loss. When addressing reduced calorie intake with patients, focus on portions and encourage physical activity such as walking more, taking the stairs, and parking further from your destination. Encourage patients to eat only when hungry and to recognize behaviors associated with overeating; eating when stressed or bored, eating after you are full, or eating too fast.

Consider Weight When Prescribing Medication

Individuals with diabetes who are gaining weight or who are having difficulty losing weight with lifestyle interventions alone may benefit from diabetes medications known to aid in weight loss. These include metformin, incretin-based therapies, or sodium glucose cotransporter 2 inhibitors.[14,18]

Discuss the carbohydrates

Carbs are macronutrients that are metabolized into sugars when digested. All foods are not equal; many foods contain carbs in varying amounts. There is insufficient evidence to support a specific carb limit for patients with diabetes; however, the amount and type of carbs matter. Consideration to the amount of carbs ingested and the patient's native insulin.[14] Patients producing a significant amount of native insulin may tolerate higher amounts of carbs compared with someone who produces very little insulin. Therefore, monitoring the amount of carbs is a key strategy for improving postprandial glucose.

Not all carbs are alike.[14] Patients with diabetes should be encouraged to choose complex carbs from vegetables, fruits, legumes, dairy products, and whole grains rather than simple carbs from processed or refined foods with added fat, sugars, and/or sodium (eg, sugary sodas, chips, white bread, and French fries). Because complex carbs take longer to digest and are usually higher in fiber content, blood sugar spikes are minimized, thus improving glycemic control.[19] Additionally, the high fiber content of complex carbs contributes to sustained satiety promoting weight loss.[19]

Strategies to Consider

1. Teach patients to recognize nutrient dense versus empty calorie carbs. Teaching patients how to read and interpret the nutrition food label before purchasing can go a long way when making healthy choices. Look for products containing protein, calcium, vitamins D, A, C, and E, iron, and fiber. The Recommended Dietary Allowances are the recommended intakes for nutrients and the percent daily value, which are listed on food labels as a requirement by the US Food and Drug Administration, determines the level of various nutrients in a serving.[20] For example, if the percent daily value for a particular nutrient (eg, fiber) is 10% or greater, that product is considered a good source of that nutrient (**Fig. 1**).Products that contain added sugar (eg, sucrose, high fructose corn syrup, corn sweetener, dextrose), saturated fat, trans fat, and/or excessive sodium (ie, >200 mg per single serving) should be limited. Therefore, patients should be encouraged to aim for products with less than 10% of the daily value of these nutrients. For better glycemic response, patients should aim for natural sources of sweetness such as fruits and some vegetables (ie, fructose), which does not rapidly increase blood sugar levels compared with table sugar (sucrose).[21]

A

Nutrition Facts

8 servings per container
Serving size   2/3 cup (55g)

Amount per serving
Calories   230

	% Daily Value*
Total Fat 8 g	**10 %**
Saturated Fat 1 g	**5 %**
Trans Fat 0 g	
Cholesterol 0 mg	**0 %**
Sodium 160 g	**7 %**
Total Carbohydrate 37 g	**13 %**
Dietary Fiber 4 g	**14 %**
Total Sugars 12 g	
Includes 10 g Added Sugars	**20 %**
Protein 3 g	
Vitamin D 2 mcg	10 %
Calcium 260 mg	20 %
Iron 8 mg	45 %
Potassium 240 mg	6 %

*The % Daily Value (DV) tells you how much a nutrient in a serving of food contributes to a daily diet. 2,000 calories a day is used for general nutrition advice.

B

Nutrition Facts

2 servings per container
Serving size   1 cup (255 g)

	Per serving		Per container	
Calories	**220**		**440**	
		% DV*		% DV*
Total Fat	5 g	**6 %**	10 g	**13 %**
Saturated Fat	2 g	**10 %**	4 g	**20 %**
Trans Fat	0 g		0 g	
Cholesterol	15 mg	**5 %**	30 mg	**10 %**
Sodium	240 mg	**10 %**	480 mg	**21 %**
Total Carb.	35 g	**13 %**	70 g	**25 %**
Dietary Fiber	6 g	**21 %**	12 g	**43 %**
Total Sugars	7 g		14 g	
Incl. Added Sugars	4 g	**8 %**	8 g	**16 %**
Protein	9 g		18 g	
Vitamin D	5 mcg	25 %	10 mcg	50 %
Calcium	200 mg	15 %	400 mg	30 %
Iron	1 mg	6 %	2 mg	10 %
Potassium	470 mg	10 %	940 mg	20 %

* The % Daily Value (DV) tells you how much a nutrient in a serving of food contributes to a daily diet. 2,000 calories a day is used for general nutrition advice.

Fig. 1. Food label reading. (*From* National Institutes of Health. *National Institute on Aging. Healthy Eating: Reading Food Labels.* Available at: https://www.nia.nih.gov/health/reading-food-labels. Accessed December 24, 2019.)

2. Encourage calorie-free and sugar-free beverages. Patients with diabetes should limit or omit sugar-sweetened beverages to decrease the risk of weight gain and risk of poor glucose control.[14] Patients should be encouraged choose water or unsweetened teas or coffees instead of sodas, fruit juices and/or sweetened teas/coffees.
3. Substitute non-nutritive sweeteners (eg, stevia or Splenda) for caloric sweeteners (eg, table sugar). When necessary, encourage patients to choose or substitute nonnutritive sweeteners for sugar to both limit calories and promote glycemic control.

Do Not Forget to Discuss Protein

When consumed with carbs, protein seems to increase insulin response, but not glucose concentrations.[14] Therefore, practitioners should encourage patients to couple carbs with protein to promote glucose uptake and avoid glucose spikes. Portion size does matter. Although protein does not significantly increase blood glucose, it still has calories; thus, eating too much can contribute to weight gain **(Table 1)**.

For individuals with diabetes and kidney disease, reducing dietary protein is not recommended to slow kidney disease progression.[14] Healthful eating patterns and weight control are the best strategies for controlling diabetes and kidney disease risk factors.

Patient Engagement

Traditionally, practitioners would take the lead in the care of their patient's diabetes by merely reviewing blood tests and making recommendations based on results.[22] These recommendations were often based on the provider's best practices, experiential knowledge, or usual care, often leaving the patient out of decisions made about their own care. Patients were often mislabeled as nonadherent or noncompliant because the recommendations did not fit their lifestyle. This approach takes the responsibility off the patient by assigning them a passive role in their health care. However, a growing body of research in diabetes care shows diabetes is better managed as a team approach with the patient taking an active role in their own health care.[22]

Patients often feel that following a diabetes diet is dreadful, requiring them to give up foods they enjoy and interfere with cultural practices. For example, African American patients who grew up in the south may be accustomed to meals high in carbs and fat (fried chicken, mac-n-cheese, candied yams, beans, and/or corn bread). Telling this patient to cut out the fried foods, pasta, and bread will be very difficult and unrealistic to follow, especially at socials or gatherings (eg, church, holidays, and Sunday

Table 1
Carb and protein combination examples

Carb Source	Protein Source
1 Slice whole wheat toast	1 Tbsp of peanut butter
1 Medium apple	Handful of almonds
1/4 Cup fresh or frozen berries	4 Oz of Plain Greek yogurt
1/2 Cup brown rice	4 oz Grilled Chicken Or Steak
½ Cup pasta	4 oz Baked chicken breast
2 Cups popcorn	1 oz Cheese stick

dinners). Rather, work with the patient to self-identify methods to modify foods. Always involve the patients; that is, after educating the patient of various foods and their impact on diabetes control, have the patient discuss what changes they can make to be more in line with food patterns that promote blood sugar control. These can include preparing yams with natural sweeteners such as honey or stevia, consuming smaller portions of mac-n-cheese and more lima beans, or preparing mac-n-cheese with whole grain pasta.

Patients must take the lead with the practitioner acting as the guide to the right food choices. This allows patients to take back control in their eating habits, thus improving their quality of life and diabetes outcomes.

Strategies to Consider

1. Educate patients rather than give facts. Many fall in the trap of just giving numbers rather than explaining what those numbers mean. You see Ms Smith, whose HbA1c has increased to 8.9% and you simply tell her, "Your HbA1c is 8.9 today. I am going to increase your Lantus from 10 units to 15 units every night. You can pick up your prescription at the front desk." All Ms Smith hears is "more insulin" rather than "your diabetes is not well-managed and we need interventions." If patients are knowledgeable about how to interpret their laboratory values, what the goals are, and what they can do, there will be better outcomes.
2. Invite patients to make decisions about the treatment plan. You may know of several effective treatments that improve weight loss and blood sugars. Instead of choosing one, tell the patient about the options, the pros and cons of each, and other patients' experiences. Once the patient has this information, ask which option will work best. Be prepared if the answer is "none of the above." This is okay too. Explore other options together to determine what works best for the patient and be prepared to have this conversation multiple times.

BREAST FEEDING

Studies suggest that breast feeding may the lower risk for T2DM and CVD development in women who breast feed. Longitudinal data from a prospective nationwide study in China examined the effects of long-term breast feeding and CVD risk. More than 289,000 postpartum women, who breast fed their infant for an average of 12 months, were followed for an 8-year period. Results from this study found that breast feeding was associated with a 10% decrease in CVD risk.[23] Although there have not been any randomized, controlled trials testing the effects of breast feeding and CVD surrogate markers such as blood pressure, diabetes, and blood lipids, moms with gestational diabetes should still be encouraged to breast feed their infants because of the many health and emotional benefits for both baby and mom.[24]

DECIPHER THE MYTHS AND THE TRUTHS ABOUT DIABETES

Again, with the massive amount of information (both true and false) at the fingertips of our patients, patients believe and share diabetes information that may not only be untrue but harmful for the patient. Therefore, it is essential for practitioners to be aware of and discuss these common myths about diabetes treatment.

Myth 1: Low-Carbohydrate Diets are Effective in Diabetes Control

The amount and type of carbs play a key role in glycemic control. Although some studies show the effect of low-carb diets (eg, Atkins, ketogenic, and vegan diets) on glycemic control and weight loss, many of these diets are difficult to maintain, affecting their impact on long-term outcomes and sustained weight loss.[25] These popular diets promote quick and easy weight loss, but patients with diabetes should be warned of quick and easy diets. The Atkins diet, which extremely restricts carbs, may increase the risk for developing hypoglycemia; especially in patients treated with insulin.[25] In contrast, diets high in fat, especially saturated and trans fat (processed meats, cheese, margarine), increase level of circulating fat and low-density cholesterol in the blood, which actually increase risk for CVD.[19]

Currently, there is no standardize recommendation for carb intake for people with diabetes. The ADA recommends that about 45% of total caloric intake come from healthful carb sources.[25] The key to glycemic control is focusing on eating healthy foods that are nutrient dense and relatively low in calories. Weight control and weight loss are key components in diabetes control.

Myth 2: Apple Cider Vinegar Cures Diabetes

Diabetes is a chronic disease that currently has no cure. Apple cider vinegar does not cure diabetes. No study has substantiated a claim for the effectiveness of apple cider vinegar in humans. Some studies, done in rats, showed some positive influence on hyperglycemia and lipid profiles, but no study has been done to test the effect of apple cider vinegar in humans.[26,27] In contrast, there is very little danger with using small amounts of apple cider vinegar in the patient population and, thus, patients can use apple cider vinegar along with their diabetic medications. However, they must take the diabetic medications, because that is the real treatment.

Myth 3: Fruit Is Healthy So You Can Eat as Much as You Want

Although fruit contains many nutrients and impact blood glucose different than table sugar, it also contains carbs, which can affect blood sugar. Like any food, fruits should be enjoyed in moderation and combined with protein-rich foods to stabilize blood sugar levels and promote satiety.

Be Prepared to Discuss Special Diets

Some patients desire to eat healthier and live a healthier life and, thus, many are turning to vegetarianism, veganism, pescatarian, and so on. Other patients have food intolerances (eg, lactose or gluten intolerance), food allergies, and/or medical conditions (eg, Crohn's disease, kidney failure); many patients with diabetes are not able to tolerate recommended foods. Patients with Crohn's disease often do not tolerate raw fruits and vegetables, dairy products, or high-fiber foods, all of which are encouraged in patients with diabetes. Therefore, this group of patients may find it very challenging to control both their diabetes and coexisting Crohn's disease.

STRATEGIES TO CONSIDER

1. Focus on foods the patient can eat. Too often, practitioners focus on what patients cannot eat, "You can't eat this, you shouldn't eat that, and you must avoid this." This practice discourages patients and leaves them feeling deprived of the foods they enjoy. Some "forbidden" foods are tolerated better than others. For example, most people with lactose intolerance are told to avoid dairy products; however, many can handle yogurts, cheese, and small portions of milk.[28] Advising patients to completely avoid key food groups puts the patients at risk for nutrient deficiency (vitamin D and calcium). Often telling a patient "you cannot have…" will actually increase desire for that food.

2. Explore and discuss patient food preferences and tolerances. Taking a few extra moments to discuss your patient's preferences and tolerances can go a long way. Use these preferences to develop with an eating plan that is, balanced, nutritious, and acceptable for the patient.

SUMMARY

The complex nature of diabetes and its management makes education of the patient challenging. Diabetes is progressive often requiring treatment adjustment over time. With the vast amount of diet information available in various media, patients with diabetes and their providers can be confused on the best strategies for diabetes management. This confusion may lead to poor adherence to treatment recommendations leading to poor outcomes.

Even though many patients with diabetes do not encounter an registered dietitian/certified diabetes educator for diabetes education and training, many will have frequent interactions with their practitioners who will play a fundamental role in the provision of diet education. Practitioners are not only responsible for providing accurate, evidenced-based dietary strategies for diabetes control, they are also responsible for involving the patients in every aspect of their care.

DISCLOSURE

The author declares no conflict of interest.

REFERENCES

1. Boyle JP, Thompson TJ, Gregg EW, et al. Projection of the year 2050 burden of diabetes in the US adult population: dynamic modeling of incidence, mortality, and prediabetes prevalence. Popul Health Metr 2010;8:29.
2. Center for Disease Prevention and Control. Adult diabetes. 2017. Available at: https://www.cdc.gov/diabetes/basics/diabetes.html. Accessed July 6, 2019.
3. Center for Disease Prevention and Control. Diabetes quick facts. 2018. Available at: https://www.cdc.gov/diabetes/basics/quick-facts.html. Accessed July 6, 2019.
4. Long AN, Dagogo-Jack S. Comorbidities of diabetes and hypertension: mechanisms and approach to target organ protection. J Clin Hypertens (Greenwich) 2011;13(4):244–51.
5. Sowers JR, Epstein M, Frohlich ED. Diabetes, hypertension, and cardiovascular disease: an update. Hypertension 2001;37:1053–9.
6. Center for Disease Prevention and Control. Who's at risk. 2017. Available at: https://www.cdc.gov/diabetes/basics/risk-factors.html. Accessed May 9, 2019.
7. Chatterjee S, Khunti K, Davies MJ. Type 2 diabetes. Lancet 2017;389(10085): 2239–51.
8. Marín-Peñalver JJ, Martín-Timón I, Sevillano-Collantes C, et al. Update on the treatment of type 2 diabetes mellitus. World J Diabetes 2016;7(17):354–95.
9. Sawyer L, Gale EA. Diet, delusion and diabetes. Diabetologia 2009;52(1):1–7.
10. Rosenfe LD. Insulin: discovering and controversy. Clin Chem 2002;48(2): 2270–88.
11. Matz R. The discovery of insulin. BMJ 2000;321(7273):1418–865.
12. Bierman EL, Albrink MY, Arky RA. Special report: principles of nutrition and dietary recommendations for patients with diabetes mellitus. Diabetes 1971;20: 633–4.

13. Mattina C, Caffrey M. Diabetes rates rise among US youth, especially minorities. Am J Manag Care 2017;23(6):205. Available at: https://www.ajmc.com/journals/evidence-based-diabetes-management/2017/june-2017/diabetes-rates-rise-among-us-youth-especially-minorities.
14. Evert AB, Boucher JL, Cypress M, et al. Nutrition therapy recommendations for the management of adults with diabetes. Diabetes Care 2013;36(11):3821–42.
15. Joslin Diabetes Center. Goals for blood sugar monitoring. 2018. Available at: https://www.joslin.org/media/23/download. Accessed July 14, 2019.
16. Robbins JM, Thatcher GE, Webb DA, et al. Nutritionist visits, diabetes classes, and hospitalization rates and charges: the Urban Diabetes Study. Diabetes Care 2008;31(4):655–60.
17. DiMaria-Ghalili RA, Mirtallo JM, Tobin BW, et al. Challenges and opportunities for nutrition education and training in the health care professions: intraprofessional and interprofessional call to action. Am J Clin Nutr 2014;99(5 Suppl):1184S–93S.
18. Effect of intensive blood-glucose control with metformin on complications in overweight patients with type 2 diabetes (UKPDS 34). UK Prospective Diabetes Study (UKPDS) Group. Lancet 1998;352(9131):854–65.
19. McArdle BS, William D, Katch F, et al. Sports and exercise nutrition. 4th edition. New York: Wolters-Kluwer, Lippincott; 2012. p. 28–31.
20. National Institute of Health Office of Dietary Supplements (UNK). Daily values. Available at: https://ods.od.nih.gov/HealthInformation/dailyvalues.aspx. Accessed July 29, 2019.
21. Shambaugh P, Worthington V, Herbert JH. Differential effects of honey, sucrose, and fructose on blood sugar levels. J Manipulative Physiol Ther 1990;13(6): 322–5.
22. Stetson B, Minges KE, Richardson CR. New directions for diabetes prevention and management in behavioral medicine. J Behav Med 2017;40(1):127–44.
23. Peters SA, Yang L, Guo Y, et al. Breastfeeding and the risk of maternal cardiovascular disease: a prospective study of 300,000 Chinese women. J Am Heart Assoc 2017;6(6) [pii:e00608].
24. American Academy of Pediatrics. Breastfeeding: breastfeeding benefits. 2018. Available at: https://www.aap.org/en-us/advocacy-and-policy/aap-health-initiatives/Breastfeeding/Pages/Benefits-of-Breastfeeding.aspx. Accessed July 17, 2019.
25. Chester B, Babu JR, Greene MW, et al. The effects of popular diets on type 2 diabetes management. Diabetes Metab Res Rev 2019;35(8):e3188.
26. Hmad Halima B, Sarra K, Jemaa Houda B, et al. Antidiabetic and antioxidant effects of apple cider vinegar on normal and streptozotocin-induced diabetic rats. Int J Vitam Nutr Res 2018;88(5–6):223–33.
27. Shishehbor F, Mansoori A, Sarkaki AR, et al. Apple cider vinegar attenuates lipid profile in normal and diabetic rats. Pak J Biol Sci 2008;11(23):2634–8.
28. National Institute of Diabetes and Digestive Kidney health. Eating, diet, & nutrition for lactose intolerance. 2018. Available at: https://www.niddk.nih.gov/health-information/digestive-diseases/lactose-intolerance/eating-diet-nutrition. Accessed July 29, 2019.

Noninsulin Therapy for Diabetes

Rebecca A. Maxson, PharmD, BCPS[a],*, Emily K. McCoy, PharmD, BCACP[b]

KEYWORDS

- Diabetes • Sodium glucose co-transport-2 inhibitors
- Glucagon-like peptide receptor agonists • Oral diabetic medications

KEY POINTS

- Glucose control and the management of comobidities in patients with T2DM are imperative in improving long term outcomes.
- Metformin remains the first line recommendation but the addition of second and third line agents now depends on patient comorbidities.
- The SGLT2 inhibitors now have data to support their use in patients with established ASCVD and/or CKD.

INTRODUCTION

For decades, metformin has been the first line noninsulin antihyperglycemic agent in the treatment of type 2 diabetes (T2DM), with the choice of additional agents being determined based on efficacy, cost, and tolerability. Before recent phase 4 cardiovascular disease (CVD) risk trials performed on the newly developed noninsulin antihyperglycemic agents, medications were added when additional hemoglobin A1c (HbA1c) lowering was required and were recommended based on individual patient factors. With this new data, both of the major diabetes guidelines (2019 American Diabetes Association's Standards of Medical Care in Diabetes and the 2019 American Association of Clinical Endocrinologists and American College of Endocrinology on the Comprehensive Type 2 Diabetes Management Algorithm) now include recommendations for preferred second agents to metformin based on benefit for special populations that is independent of HbA1c lowering.[1,2] **Table 1** contains an overview of the current guideline recommendations for noninsulin antihyperglycemic agents. What follows is a brief overview of key noninsulin agents for the treatment of T2DM (**Table 2** contains drug names by class) followed by a discussion of the literature and expert

[a] Auburn University Harrison School of Pharmacy, 1327 Walker Building, Auburn, AL 36849, USA; [b] Auburn University Harrison School of Pharmacy, 650 Clinic Drive, Suite 2100, Mobile, AL 36688, USA
* Corresponding author.
E-mail address: maxsora@auburn.edu

Physician Assist Clin 5 (2020) 153–165
https://doi.org/10.1016/j.cpha.2019.11.005
2405-7991/20/© 2019 Elsevier Inc. All rights reserved.

Table 1
Summary of 2019 American Diabetes Association's Standards of Medical Care in Diabetes and American College of Endocrinology on the comprehensive type 2 diabetes management algorithm treatment algorithms

FIRST-LINE: Metformin and Lifestyle Changes				
Add-on: Choose Based on Special Populations (See Below)				
Established Atherosclerotic CVD or CKD		Without Established Atherosclerotic CVD or CKD		
Atherosclerotic CVD Predominates	CKD or HF Predominates	Minimize Hypoglycemia	Minimize Weight Gain or Promote Weight Loss	Cost is a Major Issue
GLP-1 RA with proven CVD benefit OR SGLT2i with proven CVD benefit, if eGFR adequate	*Prefer* SGLT2i with evidence of reducing HF and/ or CKD progression if eGFR adequate OR GLP-1 RA with proven CVD benefit (only if eGFR too low, SGLT2i not tolerated)	DPP-4i OR GLP-1 RA OR SGLT2i OR TZD	GLP-1 RA with good efficacy for weight loss OR SGLT2i	Sulfonylurea OR TZD

Abbreviations: CKD, chronic kidney disease; CVD, cardiovascular disease; DPP-4i, dipeptidyl peptidase-4 inhibitor; eGFR, estimated GFR; GLP-1 RA, glucagon-like peptide-1 receptor antagonist; HF, heart failure; SGLT2i, sodium-glucose co-transport-2 inhibitor; TZD, thiazolidinedione.

Data from American Diabetes Association. Pharmacologic Approaches to Glycemic Treatment: Standards of Medical Care in Diabetes. Diabetes Care (2019). Jan;42(Supplement 1): S90-S102, Figure 9.1 and *Data from* Consensus Statement by the American Association of Clinical Endocrinologists and American College of Endocrinology on the Comprehensive Type 2 Diabetes Management Algorithm - 2019 Executive Summary. Endocrine Practice 2019;25:69-100, pp. 98 https://doi.org/10.4158/1934-2403-25.s1.1.

opinions that support the different guideline treatment recommendations for the special populations.

OVERVIEW OF MEDICATION CLASSES
Metformin

Metformin is the only agent in the biguanide class. The UKPDS 34 trial, published in 1998, provided evidence of significant improvement in all-cause and CVD mortality in the patients treated with metformin.[3,4] Metformin continues to be the first line treatment for T2DM based on both these data and its high HbA1c lowering potential, a 1.0% to 1.3% reduction on average.[1,5] Metformin lowers blood glucose via 3 mechanisms: decreases gluconeogenesis in the liver, decreases glucose absorption from the intestines, and increases peripheral uptake and utilization of glucose.[6] Common adverse drug reactions (ADRs) are primarily gastrointestinal intolerance, diarrhea, and abdominal pain. Metformin has also been associated with vitamin B_{12} deficiency and worsening neuropathic symptoms.[1] A rare but serious ADR for metformin is lactic acidosis, which is of greater risk in patients with reduced renal function. To minimize this risk, doses are adjusted based on the patient's estimated glomerular filtration rate (eGFR) and it is contraindicated at an eGFR of less than 30 mL/min/1.73 m^2.[6] Nonglycemic effects of metformin include improvement in lipids (reduction in triglycerides [TG] and low-density lipoproteins [LDL], increase high-density lipoproteins [HDL]) and blood pressure in hypertensive patients.[7,8]

Table 2
Summary of medication effects for special populations

Drug Class Generic (Brand)	CV Effects		Renal Effects	Impact On Weight	Risk of Hypoglycemia	Cost
	Atherosclerotic CVD	HF				
Biguanides Metformin (Glucophage) metformin XR (Glucophage XR)	Decrease risk	Neutral	Neutral (increased risk of lactic acidosis with eGFR < 30)	Weight neutral with possible loss	Low	Low
Sulfonylureas Glipizide (Glucotrol) Glipizide XR (Glucotrol XL) Glimepiride (Amaryl) Glyburide (Diabeta)	Neutral (possible increased risk based on older studies)	Neutral	Neutral (increased risk of hypoglycemia)	Weight gain	High	Low
Thiazolidinediones Pioglitazone (Actos) Rosiglitazone (Avandia)	Pioglitazone: possible benefit Rosiglitazone: increased risk	Increased risk	Not preferred owing to edema	Weight gain	Low	Low
Glucagon-like peptide-1 receptor agonists Dulaglutide (Trulicity) Exenatide (Bydureon) Liraglutide (Victoza, Saxenda) Lixisenatide (Adlyxin) Semaglutide (Ozempic Rybelsus)	Liraglutide, semaglutide, dulaglutide: benefit Exenatide, lixisenatide: neutral	Neutral	Liraglutide: benefit	Weight loss	Low	High
Dipeptidyl peptidase-4 inhibitors Alogliptin (Nesina) Linagliptin (Tradjenta) Saxagliptin (Onglyza) Sitagliptin (Januvia)	Neutral	Saxagliptin and alogliptin: increased risk Sitagliptin, linagliptin: Neutral	Neutral	Weight neutral	Low	High
Sodium glucose cotransporter-2 inhibitors Canagliflozin (Invokana) Dapagliflozin (Farxiga) Empagliflozin (Jardiance) Ertugliflozin (Steglatro)	Empagliflozin, canagliflozin: benefit Dapagliflozin: neutral	Benefit	Empagliflozin, canagliflozin: decreased risk of progression	Weight loss	Low	High

Abbreviations: CV, cardiovascular; eGFR, estimated glomerular filtration rate; HF, heart failure.

Sodium Glucose Cotransporter-2 Inhibitors

Sodium glucose cotransporter-2 (SGLT2) inhibitors are the newest available oral anti-hyperglycemic agents and have intermediate HbA1c lowering potential, 0.5% to 0.9% on average.[1,5] They decrease blood glucose by reducing glucose and sodium reabsorption in the proximal convoluted tubule of the kidney.[9,10] Owing to the resultant glucosuria, one of the main ADRs for SGLT2 inhibitors is genitourinary and urinary tract infections, which are more common in women. These infections can be minimized by keeping the area clean and dry.[9] Additionally, canagliflozin has a black box warning for increased risk of fractures and amputations based on the CANVAS trial.[11,12] However, the most recently published study, CREDENCE, did not show an increase in amputations in the canagliflozin group despite 5% of the study population having a history of amputations.[13] Additional ADRs include euglycemic ketoacidosis and acute kidney injury, which occurs primarily from volume depletion, and hyperkalemia.[12,14] Recently this class of medications has also been associated with Fournier gangrene.[15] Other nonglycemic effects of this class of medications include reducing blood pressure and body weight; these medications may improve TG and HDL, but they have also been associated with a slight increase in LDL.[8]

Glucagon-like Peptide-1 Receptor Antagonists

The GLP-1 receptor antagonists (RAs) also have exciting data that have expanded their use in treating T2DM. These agents reduce blood glucose via mimicking endogenous secretin. This results in enhanced postprandial insulin secretion, inhibition of glucagon, delayed gastric emptying, and increased satiety.[1] These last 2 mechanisms have led to indications for one of the agents, liraglutide, as a weight loss supplement.[16] GLP-1 RAs have high HbA1c lowering potential with an average reduction of 0.8% to 2.0% and have also been found to improve blood pressure and lower TG, LDL, and free fatty acids while also increasing HDL.[5,8,17] Although effective for glucose lowering and reducing CVD and all-cause mortality, these are primarily injectable agents requiring the patient to administer a subcutaneous injection twice daily, daily, or weekly.[9] Most patients experience transient gastrointestinal ADRs (nausea, vomiting, or diarrhea), which can sometimes lead to more serious volume depletion and acute kidney injury. Slow dose titrations and increased monitoring at the start of therapy can mitigate these risks.[9] These agents have been associated with a possible risk of acute pancreatitis. They are contraindicated in patients with a personal or family history of medullary thyroid carcinoma or multiple endocrine neoplasia type 2.[1] Although only seen in 1 study, rates of retinopathy were higher with injectable semaglutide. This result has not been seen with other GLP-1 RAs. Until further information is available, it is reasonable to avoid semaglutide in patients with preexisting retinopathy.[18]

Dipeptidyl Peptidase-4 Inhibitors

Dipeptidyl peptidase-4 (DPP-4) inhibitors have a similar mechanism of action as the GLP-1 RAs because they block the breakdown of incretin by DPP-4.[1] This results in increased native incretin effects, such as increasing postprandial insulin secretion. The DPP-4 inhibitors are generally well-tolerated and, unlike most GLP-1 RAs, are taken orally.[1,19] However, this class of medication is less efficacious in lowering HbA1c compared with the GLP-1 RAs with only an average HbA1c reduction of 0.5% to 0.9%.[1,5] Similar to the GLP-1 RAs, the DPP-4 inhibitors carry a potential risk of acute pancreatitis. DPP-4 inhibitors may lower TG, but they have little to no impact on LDL and HDL levels.[8]

Thiazolidinediones

Thiazolidinediones (TZDs) increase insulin-dependent glucose utilization in adipose and skeletal muscle tissues by activating the proliferator-activated receptor-gamma.[20] They are also highly efficacious at lowering HbA1c with an average HbA1c reduction of 0.5% to 1.4%.[1,5] Pioglitazone can lower TG, and both pioglitazone and rosiglitazone can increase HDL and LDL levels.[8] These agents are not recommended for use in patients with heart failure (HF) because they cause edema secondary to sodium and fluid retention. Additional ADRs to note include bladder cancer, anemia, and increased risk of fracture.[21]

Sulfonylureas

Sulfonylureas have been available for decades and are used widely for the treatment of T2DM because they are both cost effective and highly efficacious at lowering HbA1c, with an 0.4% to 1.2% average HbA1c reduction.[1,5] They decrease blood glucose by stimulating the pancreatic β-cells to secrete insulin.[22] As such, this class has the highest risk of causing hypoglycemia, especially in the elderly, those with decreased kidney function, or those also on insulin.[9] This class of medication also causes weight gain. Currently the second-generation agents (glipizide, glimepiride, and glyburide) are used clinically.

REVIEW OF TREATMENT BASED ON SPECIAL POPULATIONS
Atherosclerotic Cardiovascular Disease Predominates

Patients with T2DM are at significantly higher risk of cardiovascular (CV) events compared with those without diabetes. The relationship between HbA1c, CVD, and mortality is linear, and CVD risk increases approximately 16% for every 1% increase in HbA1c.[23,24] Current recommendations suggest adding to metformin, antidiabetic medications that have been proven to reduce CV risk in patients with clinical atherosclerotic CVD (ASCVD). Currently, these agents include liraglutide, injectable semaglutide, dulaglutide, empagliflozin, and canagliflozin.[1,25] These recommendations are based on large phase 4 CV effect trials that compared the new agent with placebo when added to standard of care in patients with risk for CVD. For all trials, the primary end point was a composite of CV death, nonfatal myocardial infarction, and nonfatal stroke. **Table 3** provides a summary of the key baseline characteristics, the primary outcome results, and any statistically significant secondary outcomes.

CV effects of the GLP-1 RAs liraglutide, semaglutide, exenatide, lixisenatide, and dulaglutide have been evaluated in several trials (LEADER, SUSTAIN-6, EXSCEL, ELIXA, REWIND, respectively). Liraglutide and semaglutide were shown to reduce CV events in patients with established CVD, whereas dulaglutide demonstrated CV benefit in both primary and secondary prevention patients.[18,26,27] There was a significant decrease seen in the secondary outcomes of CV death and all-cause mortality in the LEADER trial, while SUSTAIN-6 and REWIND demonstrated a reduction in the secondary outcome of stroke.[18,26,27] Exenatide, lixisenatide, and oral semaglutide have been found to have a neutral CV effect compared with placebo.[28–30] The findings from the CV trials with GLP-1 RAs suggest that these agents lower CV risk by an anti-atherosclerotic mechanism.[24]

Recent evidence indicates that SGLT2 inhibitors also have cardioprotective effects in high-risk patients with T2DM. Empagliflozin, canagliflozin, and most recently dapagliflozin have been studied in patients with T2DM and established CVD or multiple risk factors. Empagliflozin and canagliflozin were found to significantly decrease the primary composite CV end point, and empagliflozin also decreased the secondary end

Table 3
Summary data for CVD, HF, and CKD effects of recommended antidiabetic agents

Medication	GLP-1 RAs						SGLT2 Inhibitors			
	Liraglutide	Semaglutide Injectable	Semaglutide Oral	Dulaglutide	Exenatide Weekly	Lixisenatide	Empagliflozin	Canagliflozin	Canagliflozin	Dapagliflozin
Trial	LEADER[26]	SUSTAIN-6[18]	PIONEER-6[28]	REWIND[27]	EXSCEL[29]	ELIXA[30]	EMPA-REG[31,43]	CANVAS[11]	CREDENCE[13]	DECLARE-TIMI 58[32]
No. of patients	9340	3297	3183	9901	14,752	6068	7020	10,142	4401	17,610
Median follow-up (y)	3.8	2.1	1.3	5.4	3.2	2.1	3.1	2.4	2.62	4.2
Mean age (y)	64	64	66	66	62	60	63	63.3	63	64
Baseline HbA1c (%)	8.7	8.7	8.2	7.3	8.0	7.7	8.1	8.2	8.3	8.3
Atherosclerotic CVD (%)	81	72	85	31.5	73	100	100	72		41
eGFR (mL/min/1.73 m²)	41% 60–89 20% 30–59 2.4% < 30	30% ≥ 90 41% 60–89 25% 30–59 2.7% 15–29 0.4% ESKD		22% < 60	29% > 90 49% 60–89 21% 30–59 0.1% < 30	Avg eGFR 76	21% ≥ 90 52% 60–89 26% < 60	Avg eGFR 76	4.8% ≥ 90 35% 60–89 28.8% 45–59 27% 30–44 3.8% 15–29 0.1% < 15	7% < 60
UACR				35% > 3.39 (mg/mmol)		Avg 10 (mg/g)	59.5% < 30 28% 30–300 11% > 300 (mg/g)	Avg 12.3 mg/g 22.6% microalbuminuria 7.6% macroalbuminuria	0.7% < 30 11% 30–300 76% 300–3000 11% > 3000 (mg/g)	

Outcomes HR (95% CI)								
Primary CV outcome	0.87 (0.78-0.97)	0.74 (0.58-0.95)	0.79 (0.57-1.11)	0.88 (0.79-0.99)	1.02 (0.89-1.17)	0.86 (0.74-0.99)	0.86 (0.75-0.97)	0.93 (0.84-1.03)
CV death	0.78 (0.66-0.93)	0.98 (0.65-1.48)	0.49 (0.27-0.92)	0.91 (0.78-1.06)	0.98 (0.78-1.22)	0.62 (0.49-0.77)	0.87 (0.72-1.06)	0.98 (0.82-1.17)
Myocardial infarction	0.86 (0.73-1.00)	0.74 (0.51-1.08)	1.18 (0.73-1.90)	0.96 (0.79-1.15)	1.03 (0.87-1.22)	0.87 (0.70-1.09)	0.89 (0.73-1.09)	0.89 (0.77-1.01)
Stroke	0.86 (0.71-1.06)	0.61 (0.38-0.99)	0.74 (0.35-1.57)	0.76 (0.62-0.94)	1.12 (0.79-1.58)	1.18 (0.89-1.56)	0.87 (0.74-1.01)	1.01 (0.84-1.21)
All-cause mortality	0.85 (0.74-0.97)	1.05 (0.74-1.50)	0.51 (0.31-0.84)	0.90 (0.80-1.01)	0.86 (0.77-0.97)	0.68 (0.57-0.82)	0.87 (0.74-1.01)	0.93 (0.82-1.04)
HF hospitalizations	0.87 (0.73-1.05)	1.11 (0.77-1.61)	0.86 (0.48-1.55)	0.93 (0.77-1.22)	0.96 (0.75-1.23)	0.65 (0.50-0.85)	0.67 (0.52-0.87)	0.73 (0.61-0.88)
Renal outcomes	0.78 (0.67-0.92)[a]	0.64 (0.46-0.98)[b]	0.85 (0.77-0.93)[c]	0.85 (0.73-0.98)[d]	Not clinically significant change in UACR between 2 groups	0.61 (0.53-0.70)[e] 0.54 (0.40-0.75)[f]	0.73 (0.67-0.79)[g] 0.60 (0.47-0.77)[h] 0.70 (0.59-0.82)[i] 0.60 (0.48-0.76)[j] 0.68 (0.45-0.80)[k]	0.53 (0.43-0.66)[l]

Abbreviations: CI, confidence interval; UACR, urine albumin: creatinine ratio; ESKD, end-stage kidney disease.

a Nephropathy (macroalbuminuria, doubling of serum creatinine and eGFR of 45 or less, ESRD, or death owing to renal disease).
b New or worsening nephropathy (macroalbuminuria, doubling of serum creatinine and an eGFR of 45 or less, or ESRD).
c New macroalbuminuria, a 30% or greater decrease in the eGFR, or chronic renal replacement therapy.
d A 40% decrease in the eGFR, renal replacement therapy, renal death, or macroalbuminuria.
e Incident or worsening nephropathy.
f Post hoc renal composite outcome.
g Progression of albuminuria.
h A 40% decrease in eGFR, renal replacement therapy or renal death.
i Primary renal composite.
j Secondary outcome: doubling serum creatinine.
k Secondary outcome: ESRD.
l A 40% or greater decrease in eGFR to less than 60, ESRD, death from renal causes.

points of CV death and all-cause mortality.[11,31] The decrease in mortality was seen very early in the trial and persisted throughout the duration of the trial.[31] However, the majority of the patients in both trials had established CVD. Dapagliflozin has been studied in more of a primary prevention population, and although dapagliflozin was shown to not worsen CV risk, it also did not improve primary CV outcomes.[32] The early and sustained benefits seen with the SGLT2 inhibitors suggest the CV benefits are secondary to hemodynamic factors.[24]

The DPP-4 inhibitors saxaglipitin, alogliptin, sitagliptin, and linagliptin have also been evaluated for CV safety.[33–36] None of these agents have been found to increase risk for adverse CV events, CV mortality or all-cause mortality, nor have they demonstrated CV benefit; however, an increase in HF risk was seen and is discussed elsewhere in this article. The CV safety of sulfonylureas has been questioned, as observational studies have suggested an increase in CV risk.[24] Meta-analyses evaluating CV risk have been conflicting, with some analyses suggesting elevated CV risk and others suggesting no difference exists.[37–39] The variability in results likely lies in the heterogeneity of the available data and study design. The recent CAROLINA trial compared the CV safety of linagliptin and glimepiride in patients with T2DM and either high CV risk or established CVD. Investigators found no significant differences in CV events, although a higher risk of hypoglycemia and weight gain was found in the sulfonylurea arm of the trial.[40]

TZDs have also had safety concerns regarding CV risk. Rosiglitazone has been associated with increase CV risk leading to it being withdrawn from the European market and having restricted use in the United States.[24] Two trials have evaluated the safety of pioglitazone. The Prospective Pioglitazone Clinical Trial In Macrovascular Events (PROactive) trial demonstrated no significant difference in the primary composite end point, but pioglitazone use did reduce the secondary end point of all-cause mortality, nonfatal myocardial infarction, and stroke ($P = .027$).[41] Pioglitazone has also been associated with a lower risk of stroke or myocardial infarction in patients with recent stroke or transient ischemic attack with insulin resistance but without T2DM.[42]

Chronic Kidney Disease or Heart Failure Predominates

Several of the CV trials mentioned in the previous section also had kidney and HF hospitalization outcomes as secondary end points (see **Table 3**). SGLT2 inhibitors have demonstrated significant reductions in HF hospitalizations compared with placebo in both patients with and without HF at baseline.[11,32,43] Based on this promising data, the SGLT2 inhibitors are now being studied in HF patients who do not have T2DM. The GLP-1 RA trials did not show statistically significant lowering of HF hospitalizations.[18,26–30] Therefore the recent guidelines recommend canagliflozin or empagliflozin over GLP-1RAs (if tolerated) for patients with HF.[1,2]

In these same trials, various kidney outcomes were also included as secondary outcomes. Although the GLP-1 RA trials showed statistically significant reductions in the various kidney outcomes studied, there were very few patients with CKD or albuminuria included in these trials.[18,26–30] However, the trials for canagliflozin (CANVAS) and empagliflozin (EMPA-REG) did include a significant number of patients with preexisting CKD and showed clinically significant reductions in the renal outcomes (see **Table 3**).[11,31,43] In comparison, the DECLARE TIMI 58 trial showed significant reductions in kidney outcomes, but only 7% of the population had an eGFR of less than 60 mL/min/1.73 m[2].[32] Thus, the guidelines prefer canagliflozin or empagliflozin for patients with CKD; the GLP-1 RAs with CV benefit are recommended as alternatives for patients who do not tolerate SGLT2 inhibitors or have an eGFR that is too low.[1]

Based on the CREDENCE Trial, canaglifozin is the first SGLT2 inhibitor to obtain a US Food and Drug Administration indication for decreasing the risk of ESRD, doubling the serum creatinine, CV death, and HF hospitalization and doubling the serum creatinine in patients with diabetes and albuminuria.[12] The CREDENCE trial, which included patients with an eGFR of less than 60 mL/min/1.73 m^2, showed kidney benefits in all eGFR prespecified subgroups: an eGFR of 45 to less than 60 mL/min/1.73 m^2 (29% of patients) and 30 to less than 45 mL/min/1.73 m^2 (30% of patients).[13] Based on these data, the updated US Food and Drug Administration prescribing information for canagliflozin includes the following dose recommendations for patients with CKD: for an eGFR of 60 or greater, 100 mg/d with possible increase to 300 mg/d for additional glycemic control; for an eGFR of 45 to less than 60, 100 mg/d; for an eGFR of 30 to less than 45 with an albuminuria of greater than 300 mg/d, 100 mg/d; and contraindicated if on dialysis.[10,12]

Compelling Need to Minimize Hypoglycemia

Hypoglycemia (defined as a blood glucose of <70 mg/dL) is associated with an increase in CV events, all-cause mortality, increased patient fear, and decreased quality of life.[44] Risk factors for hypoglycemia include older age, longer duration of diabetes, cognitive impairment, impaired kidney or hepatic function, hypoglycemia unawareness, alcohol use, and polypharmacy.[1] Current guidelines recommend adding a DPP-4 inhibitor, SGLT2 inhibitor, GLP-1 RA, or TZD to metformin therapy if the desire is to minimize the risk of hypoglycemia.[1,25] The risk of hypoglycemia with SGLT2 inhibitors is low, because the effect on glucose elimination is proportional to the glycemic load; higher glucose levels result in greater urinary elimination, whereas glucose elimination is negligible in instances of mild to modest hyperglycemia.[24] GLP-1 RAs and DPP-4 inhibitors both cause glucose-dependent insulin secretion, leading to a low risk of hypoglycemia as monotherapy. However, the risk of hypoglycemia increases if these agents are combined with sulfonylureas.[24]

Insulin secretagogues such as sulfonylureas, which cause glucose-independent insulin secretion, and insulin are associated with hypoglycemia and should be avoided if possible in patients when this is a concern.[1,25] If sulfonylureas are used, consideration should be given to using either glipizide or glimepiride as these agents have a lower risk of hypoglycemia compared with glyburide.[1,25] Patients should be counseled to administer these medications 30 minutes before a meal to minimize the risk of hypoglycemia.

Minimize Weight Gain and Promote Weight Loss

Obesity is a common risk factor for the development and progression of T2DM. Peripheral insulin resistance with T2DM develops as a result of ectopic fat deposition in the liver, muscle, and pancreatic β-cells, which can lead to a decrease in β-cell function, islet inflammation, and β-cell death.[45,46] A modest weight loss of even 5% can improve glucose control, decrease diabetes-associated complications, and improve CV risk factors.[45,47,48] Metformin is weight neutral and may promote slight weight loss; the mechanism behind this, although not fully understood, is possibly related to the anorectic effects.[45]

SGLT2 inhibitors and GLP-1 RAs are both associated with weight loss and are preferred after metformin therapy for patients in whom weight loss is desired.[1,25] SGLT2 inhibitors cause weight loss primarily through glucosuria, with 60 to 80 g of glucose eliminated per day, as well as through fluid loss owing to osmotic diuresis.[24,45] Clinical trials with the SGLT2 inhibitors have demonstrated a weight loss of 0.9 to

2.6 kg, and weight loss with this class of medications decreases total body fat, waist circumference, visceral adiposity, and central obesity.[45,49] GLP-1 RAs cause weight loss by delaying gastric emptying, decreasing appetite, and increasing satiety, and these agents are associated with a dose-dependent weight loss of 0.8 to 6.9 kg.[45,50] Studies have shown a reduction in visceral and subcutaneous fat, as well as waist circumference with GLP-1 RAs.[51]

DPP-4 inhibitors are considered weight neutral, with a weight range change of −0.9 to +1.1 kg, and these agents may be used after an SGLT2 inhibitor if the patient is not already on a GLP-1 RA and additional glucose control is needed.[1,45] Sulfonylureas, meglitinides, and TZDs are all associated with weight gain and should be avoided when possible in patients who are overweight or obese. Of these, TZDs are likely to cause the most weight gain (2.3–4.3 kg) through fluid retention and redistribution of adipose tissue, while sulfonylureas may cause a weight gain of up to 2.3 to 2.7 kg.[45]

Cost Is a Major Issue

Based on the 2017 National Diabetes Statistics Report from the Centers for Disease Control and Prevention, the prevalence of diagnosed diabetes is influenced by level of education, which is a marker of socioeconomic status.[52] The highest prevalence of diabetes (12.6%) occurs in patients who did not finish high school, with 9.5% in patients with a high school education and 7.2% in patients with more than high school education. Potentially a significant portion of the 23 million Americans with diabetes have cost as a major concern in managing their disease. The least expensive noninsulin agents are metformin, TZDs, and sulfonylureas. After starting metformin, if additional HbA1c lowering is needed or the patient does not tolerate metformin, either a sulfonylurea or TZD may be added. As described elsewhere in this article, sulfonylureas have the greatest risk of hypoglycemia and so might be less preferred for patients with hypoglycemia unawareness. TZDs can cause edema making them less preferred for patients with HF or CKD.[1]

SUMMARY

Glucose control and the management of comorbidities in patients with T2DM are imperative in improving long term outcomes. Metformin remains the first line recommendation for treatment of T2DM, but the addition of second and third line agents depends largely on patient comorbidities.[1,2] With the high incidence of atherosclerotic CVD in patients with T2DM, recent data provide strong support for CV risk reduction with the use of empagliflozin, canagliflozin, liraglutide, and semaglutide in patients with established atherosclerotic CVD; dulaglutide has the strongest evidence for CV benefit in a primary prevention population. These studies also provide evidence for improving outcomes in patients with HF and CKD, 2 additional high-risk T2DM populations, when the SGLT2 inhibitors, canagliflozin, and empagliflozin are used. Providers should take the patient's weight, risk of hypoglycemia, and ability to pay for medications into consideration, as well when adding a second-line therapy to metformin. The treatment of T2DM remains a multifaceted approach and ongoing clinical trials will continue to provide guidance on optimal medication use in this patient population.

DISCLOSURE

Dr R.A. Maxson and Dr E.K. McCoy have nothing to disclose regarding commercial or financial conflicts of interest.

REFERENCES

1. American Diabetes Association. Standards of medical care in diabetes- 2019. Diabetes Care 2019;42(Supplement 1):S1–193.
2. Garber AJ, Abrahamson MJ, Barzilay JI, et al. Consensus Statement by the American Association of Clinical Endocrinologists and American College of Endocrinology on the Comprehensive Type 2 Diabetes Management Algorithm – 2019 Executive Summary. Endocr Pract 2019;25:69–100.
3. UK Prospective Diabetes Study (UKPDS) Group. Effect of intensive blood-glucose control with metformin on complications in overweight patients with type 2 diabetes (UKPDS 34). Lancet 1998;352(9131):854–65.
4. Maruther NM, Tseng E, Hufless S, et al. Diabetes medications as monotherapy or metformin-based combination therapy for type 2 diabetes. Ann Intern Med 2016; 164(11):740–51.
5. George C, Bruijn L. Management of blood glucose with noninsulin therapies in type 2 diabetes. Am Fam Physician 2015;92:27–34.
6. Glucophage [package insert]. Princeton (NJ): Bristol-Myers Squibb Company. Available at: https://www.accessdata.fda.gov/drugsatfda_docs/label/2017/02035 7s037s039,021202s021s023lbl.pdf. Accessed July 19, 2019.
7. Anabtawi A, Miles JM. Metformin: nonglycemic effects and potential novel indications. Endocr Pract 2016;22(8):999–1007.
8. Rosenblit PD. Common medications used by patients with type 2 diabetes mellitus: what are their effects on the lipid profile? Cardiovasc Diabetol 2016;15:95.
9. Roussel R, Lorraine J, Rodriguez A, et al. Overview of data concerning safe use of antihyperglycemic medications in type 2 diabetes mellitus and chronic kidney disease. Adv Ther 2015;32:1029–64.
10. Bakris G. Major advancements in slowing diabetic kidney disease progression: focus on SGLT2 inhibitors. Am J Kidney Dis 2019. https://doi.org/10.1053/j.ajkd.2019.05.009.
11. Neal B, Perkovic V, Mahaffey KW, et al. Canagliflozin and cardiovascular and renal outcomes in type 2 diabetes. N Engl J Med 2017;377:644–57.
12. Invokana [package insert]. Titusville (NJ): Janssen Pharmaceuticals, Inc.; 2019. Available at: http://www.janssenlabels.com/package-insert/product-monograph/prescribing-information/INVOKANA-pi.pdf. Accessed Oct 16, 2019.
13. Perkovic V, Jardine MJ, Neal B, et al. Canagliflozin and renal outcomes in type 2 diabetes and nephropathy. N Engl J Med 2019;380:2295–306.
14. Farxiga [package insert]. Wilmington (DE): AstraZeneca Pharmaceuticals LP; 2016. Available at: https://www.accessdata.fda.gov/drugsatfda_docs/label/2017/202293s012lbl.pdf#page=29. Accessed July 19, 2019.
15. Bersoff-Matcha SJ, Chamberlain C, Cao C, et al. Fournier gangrene associated with sodium-glucose cotransporter-2 inhibitors: a review of spontaneous postmarketing cases. Ann Intern Med 2019. https://doi.org/10.7326/M19-0085.
16. Saxenda [package insert]. Plainsboro (NJ): Novo Nordis, Inc.; 2014. Available at: https://www.novo-pi.com/saxenda.pdf. Accessed July 19, 2019.
17. Chilton R, Wyatt J, Nandish S, et al. Cardiovascular comorbidities of type 2 diabetes mellitus: defining the potential of glucagon like peptide-1-based therapies. Am J Med 2011;124:S35–53.
18. Marso SP, Bain SC, Consoli A, et al. Semaglutide and cardiovascular outcomes in patients with type 2 diabetes. N Engl J Med 2016;375:1834–44.

19. Abe M, Okada K. DPP-4 inhibitors in diabetic patients with chronic kidney disease and end-stage kidney disease on dialysis in clinical practice. Contrib Nephrol 2015;185:98–115.

20. Actos [package insert]. Deerfield, IL: Takeda Pharmaceuticals America, Inc.. Available at: http://general.takedapharm.com/content/file.aspx?filetypecode=actospi&cacheRandomizer=d3b4d95a-598b-4eb0-bffd-540f11ed02fe. Accessed July 19, 2019.

21. Neumiller JJ, Alicic RZ, Tuttle KR. Therapeutic considerations for antihyperglycemic agents in diabetic kidney disease. J Am Soc Nephrol 2017;28:2263–74.

22. Amaryl [package insert]. Bridgewater, NJ: Sanofi-Aventis U.S. LLC. Available at: http://products.sanofi.us/Amaryl/Amaryl.pdf. Accessed July 19, 2019.

23. Khaw KT, Wareham N, Bingham S, et al. Association of hemoglobin A1c with cardiovascular disease and mortality in adults: the European prospective investigation into cancer in Norfolk. Ann Intern Med 2004;141:413–20.

24. Paneni F, Luscher TF. Cardiovascular protection in the treatment of type 2 diabetes: a review of clinical trial results across drug classes. Am J Cardiol 2017;120(suppl):S17–27.

25. Davies MJ, D'Alessio DA, Fradkin J, et al. Management of hyperglycemia in type 2 diabetes, 2018. A consensus report by the American Diabetes Association (ADA) and the European Association for the Study of Diabetes (EASD). Diabetes Care 2018;41(12):2669–701.

26. Marso SP, Daniels GH, Brown-Frandsen K, et al. Liraglutide and cardiovascular outcomes in type 2 diabetes. N Engl J Med 2016;375:311–22.

27. Gerstein HC, Colhoun HM, Dagenais GR, et al. Dulaglutide and cardiovascular outcomes in type 2 diabetes (REWIND): a double-blind, randomized placebo controlled trial. Lancet 2019;394:121–30.

28. Husain M, Birkenfeld AL, Donsmark M, et al. Oral semaglutide and cardiovascular outcomes in patients with type 2 diabetes. N Engl J Med 2019;2019. https://doi.org/10.1056/NEJMoa1901118.

29. Holman RR, Bethel MA, Mentz RJ, et al. Effects of once-weekly exenatide on cardiovascular outcomes in type 2 diabetes. N Engl J Med 2017;377:1228–39.

30. Pfeffer MA, Claggett B, Diaz R, et al. Lixisenatide in patients with type 2 diabetes and acute coronary syndrome. N Engl J Med 2015;373:2247–57.

31. Zinman B, Wanner C, Lachin JM, et al. Empagliflozin, cardiovascular outcomes, and mortality in type 2 diabetes. N Engl J Med 2015;373:2117–28.

32. Wiviott SD, Raz I, Bonaca MP, et al. Dapagliflozin and cardiovascular outcomes in type 2 diabetes. N Engl J Med 2019;380:347–57.

33. Green JB, Bethel MA, Armstrong PW, et al. Effect of sitagliptin on cardiovascular outcomes in type 2 diabetes. N Engl J Med 2015;373:232–42.

34. Rosenstock J, Perkovic V, Johansen OE, et al. Effect of linagliptin vs placebo on major cardiovascular events in adults with type 2 diabetes and high cardiovascular and renal risk: the CARMELINA randomized clinical trial. JAMA 2019;321(1):69–79.

35. Scirica BM, Bhatt DL, Braunwald E, et al. Saxagliptin and cardiovascular outcomes in type 2 diabetes. N Engl J Med 2013;369:1317–26.

36. Zannad F, Cannon CP, Cushman WC, et al. Heart failure and mortality outcomes in patients with type 2 diabetes taking alogliptin versus placebo in EXAMINE: a multicenter, randomized, double-blind trial. Lancet 2015;385:2067–76.

37. Azoulay L, Suissa S. Sulfonylureas and the risk of cardiovascular events and death: a methodological meta-regression analysis of the observational studies. Diabetes Care 2017;40:706–14.

38. Powell WR, Christiansen CL, Miller DR. Meta-analysis of sulfonylurea therapy on long-term risk of mortality and cardiovascular events compared to other oral glucose-lowering treatments. Diabetes Ther 2018;9:1431–40.
39. Rados DV, Pinto LC, Remonti LR, et al. The association between sulfonylurea use and all-cause and cardiovascular mortality: a meta-analysis with trial sequential analysis of randomized clinical trials. PLoS Med 2016;13(4):e1001992.
40. American Diabetes Association 2019 Scientific Sessions. Cardiovascular outcome study of linagliptin versus glimepiride in patients with type 2 diabetes (CAROLINA). Presented San Francisco, June 10, 2019.
41. Dormandy JA, Charbonnel B, Eckland DJ, et al. Secondary prevention of macrovascular events in patients with type 2 diabetes in the PROactive Study (PROspective pioglitAzone Clinical Trial In macro-Vascular Events): a randomised controlled trial. Lancet 2005;366:1279–89.
42. Kernan WN, Viscoli CM, Furie KL, et al. Pioglitazone after ischemic stroke or transient ischemic attack. N Engl J Med 2016;374:1321–31.
43. Wanner C, Inzucchi SE, Lachin JM, et al. Empagliflozin and progression of kidney disease in type 2 diabetes. N Engl J Med 2016;375:323–34.
44. International Hypoglycaemia Study Group. Minimizing hypoglycemia in diabetes. Diabetes Care 2015;38(8):1583–91.
45. Apovian CM, Okemah J, O'Neil PM. Body weight considerations in the management of type 2 diabetes. Adv Ther 2019;36:44–58.
46. Skyler JS, Bakris GL, Bonifacio E, et al. Differentiation of diabetes by pathophysiology, natural history, and prognosis. Diabetes 2017;66:241–55.
47. Scheen AJ, Van Gaal LF. Combating the dual burden: therapeutic targeting of common pathways in obesity and type 2 diabetes. Lancet Diabetes Endocrinol 2014;2:911–22.
48. Wing RR, Lang W, Wadden TA, et al. Benefits of modest weight loss in improving cardiovascular risk factors in overweight and obese individuals with type 2 diabetes. Diabetes Care 2011;34:1481–6.
49. Pinto LR, Rados DV, Remonti LR, et al. Efficacy of SGLT2 inhibitors in glycemic control, weight loss and blood pressure reduction: a systematic review and meta-analysis. Diabetol Metab Syndr 2015;7(Suppl 1):A58.
50. Brown E, Wilding JPH, Barber TM, et al. Weight loss variability with SGLT2 inhibitors and GLP-1 receptor agonists in type 2 diabetes mellitus and obesity: mechanistic possibilities. Obes Rev 2019;6:816–28.
51. Ryan D, Acosta A. GLP-1 receptor agonists: nonglycemic clinical effects in weight loss and beyond. Obesity (Silver Spring) 2015;23(6):1119–29.
52. Centers for Disease Control and Prevention. National diabetes statistics report: estimates of diabetes and its burden in the United States, 2017. Atlanta (GA): U.S. Department of Health and Human Services, Centers for Disease Control and Prevention; 2017. Available at: https://www.cdc.gov/diabetes/pdfs/data/statistics/national-diabetes-statistics-report.pdf. Accessed Jul 19, 2019.

Pens and Needles
Insulin Therapy for Diabetes

Sarah V. Cogle, PharmD, BCCCP[a],*,
Amber M. Hutchison, PharmD, BCPS, BCGP[b]

KEYWORDS

• Insulin • Hyperglycemia • Type 2 diabetes mellitus • Type 1 diabetes mellitus

KEY POINTS

- Insulin therapy is required in patients with type 1 diabetes mellitus.
- Insulin can be used in combination with metformin and many other oral agents to manage type 2 diabetes mellitus.
- Basal insulin, combined with prandial insulin, is a commonly used and effective regimen for many patients with type 2 diabetes mellitus.

INTRODUCTION

Insulin has been a cornerstone of treatment of hyperglycemia since its discovery in 1921.[1] At present there are a variety of insulin formulations, including rapid-acting, short-acting, intermediate-acting, and long-acting insulins. These products are now available in multiple formulations, including traditional vials, prefilled pens, cartridges for reusable pens, and inhaled insulin. Although many newer products are more expensive, there is a wide range of price points for insulin products, giving practitioners and patients more therapeutic options than ever.

AVAILABLE INSULIN PRODUCTS

Insulin is commercially available in rapid-acting and short-acting forms, which are generally used as prandial insulin, and also in intermediate-acting or long-acting forms used for basal therapy (**Tables 1** and **2**). Insulin products have traditionally come in a standard 100 units/mL (or U-100) concentration, but multiple concentrated insulin products are now available in the United States. Concentrated insulin allows higher doses of insulin to be administered in smaller volumes. Regular insulin U-500 is 5 times more concentrated than the typical U-100 regular insulin. Regular U-500 has a longer onset and extended duration of action; therefore, it may behave more as an intermediate-acting insulin.[2,3] Long-acting insulins, including glargine and degludec,

[a] Pharmacy Practice Department, Auburn University Harrison School of Pharmacy, 4201G Walker Building, Auburn, AL 36849, USA; [b] Pharmacy Practice Department, Auburn University Harrison School of Pharmacy, 1321 B Walker Building, Auburn, AL 36849, USA
* Corresponding author.
E-mail address: sev0002@auburn.edu

Physician Assist Clin 5 (2020) 167–176
https://doi.org/10.1016/j.cpha.2019.11.006
2405-7991/20/© 2019 Elsevier Inc. All rights reserved.

Table 1
Prandial insulin products

Generic Name	Brand Names	Available Dosage Forms	Timing of Administration:
Rapid Acting			
Aspart	Novolog, Fiasp	U-100 vial, U-100 prefilled pen, U-200 prefilled pen, U-100 cartridge	Fiasp: at beginning of meal or within 20 min after a meal Novolog: within 5–10 min before a meal
Lispro	Humalog, Admelog	U-100 vial, U-100 prefilled pen, U-100 cartridge	Humalog: within 5–10 min before a meal Admelog: within 15 min before a meal or immediately after a meal
Glulisine	Apidra	U-100 prefilled pen, U-100 vial	Within 15 min before a meal or within 20 min after starting a meal
Inhaled insulin (technosphere inhaled insulin)	Afrezza	4-unit, 8-unit, and 12-unit single-use cartridges Inhaler device must be replaced every 15 d	At the beginning of a meal
Short Acting			
Human regular	Humulin R, Novolin R, Novolin R ReliOn	U-100 vial	30 min before meals
Human regular (concentrated) *Delayed onset and longer duration; may behave more like intermediate-acting insulin*	Humulin R U-500	U-500 vial, U-500 prefilled pen	30 min before meals Must use U-500 insulin syringe

Data from Refs.[2–4,21–27]

are available in more concentrated forms. U-300 glargine has a longer duration than traditional U-100 glargine, although it may be less effective per unit.[2] Lispro is also now available in a U-200 prefilled pen.[4] With the exception of U-500 regular insulin, concentrated insulin products are available only in prefilled pens in order to improve patient safety by decreasing the risk of dosing errors.[2]

INSULIN THERAPY IN THE OUTPATIENT SETTING
Indications for Use

Type 1 diabetes mellitus (T1DM) is characterized by low to no beta-cell function and requires insulin therapy. Without the provision of insulin therapy, patients with T1DM

Table 2		
Basal insulin products		
Generic Name	**Brand Names**	**Available Dosage Forms**
Intermediate Acting		
NPH	Humulin N, Novolin N, Novolin N ReliOn	U-100 vials, U-100 prefilled pens
Long Acting		
Degludec	Tresiba	U-100 vial, U-100 prefilled pen, U-200 prefilled pen
Detemir	Levemir	U-100 vial, U-100 prefilled pen
Glargine	Lantus, Basaglar, Toujeo	U-100 vial, U-100 prefilled pen, U-300 prefilled pen

Abbreviation: NPH, neutral protamine hagedorn.
Data from Refs.[2,28–34]

experience substantial hyperglycemia, hypertriglyceridemia, ketoacidosis, and tissue breakdown, which lead to hospitalization and death. The American Diabetes Association (ADA) 2019 Standards of Care suggests the use of multiple daily injections of prandial and basal insulin or continuous subcutaneous insulin infusions for patients with T1DM. Rapid-acting insulin products are also recommended in this patient population in order to decrease the risk of hypoglycemia. Insulin pumps may also be appropriate in this population, as described later.[2]

In contrast, oral metformin is the first-line agent for the treatment of type 2 diabetes mellitus (T2DM), whereas other oral agents and insulin therapy can be considered as second-line options. Although oral agents are often preferred by patients, it is common for patients with T2DM to eventually require insulin therapy, particularly if the disease is present for many years and the effectiveness of oral agents has waned. The ADA suggests insulin therapy should be normalized and not treated as a threat to patients as a consequence of nonadherence with other agents.[2] Normalizing the use of insulin could help some patients overcome barriers of resistance to this therapy.

The ADA recommends the use of early insulin in patients with T2DM who show signs of catabolism (including weight loss), have symptomatic hyperglycemia, a hemoglobin A1c level greater than 10%, or very increased blood glucose levels (>300 mg/dL). Basal insulin therapy is intended to curb the production of glucose in the liver and maintain euglycemia throughout a 24-hour period. Intermediate-acting neutral protamine Hagedorn (NPH) insulin or a long-acting insulin product can be used as basal insulin therapy. These agents may be given in combination with a variety of other medications in patients who have an A1c level greater than 1.5% more than target, or in patients who have not achieved target A1c after 3 months of metformin monotherapy, provided the patient does not have atherosclerotic cardiovascular disease or severe chronic kidney disease. Many patients eventually require prandial insulin, which is given in addition to basal insulin and administered before meals to cover increases in blood glucose levels related to carbohydrate intake.[2]

Insulin Dosing

In patients with T1DM, insulin requirements are generally weight based, with a dose of 0.4 to 1 units/kg/d. Typically 50% of the daily dose is administered as basal insulin, with the remaining 50% given as prandial insulin being divided over 3 meals.[2]

In patients with T2DM, basal insulin therapy is commonly added to metformin or other oral medications. Typically, basal insulin therapy for T2DM is initiated at 10 units/d (or 0.1–0.2 units/kg/d) and titrated based on patient response. NPH or long-acting insulin products both control fasting blood glucose, but some meta-analyses have found long-acting products (including glargine or detemir) are associated with lower rates of symptomatic and nocturnal hypoglycemia compared with NPH insulin.[2,5,6] In addition, some trials have found that the use of concentrated or ultra–long-acting insulin products, including U-300 glargine or degludec, in combination with oral agents, achieved glycemic targets with a lower rate of hypoglycemia compared with traditional U-100 glargine combined with oral agents.[7–9] Although longer-acting or concentrated products may offer advantages, these products generally are more expensive than NPH insulin. The risk/benefit profile along with cost must be considered and individualized to the patient when selecting an insulin regimen.

Combination Therapy

Several products containing both a basal and prandial component are available (**Table 3**), which can be advantageous for many patients because these therapies typically require fewer total daily injections and may be more cost-effective than purchasing multiple individual insulin products. Combination insulins are generally dosed twice daily, with each dose intended to cover 2 meals or a meal and a snack.

In patients receiving basal insulin therapy who have controlled fasting blood glucose levels but with an A1c level that continues to exceed the target range (or if the dose of basal insulin therapy is >0.5 units/kg/d), combination injectable therapy can be considered. In general, the therapy added is a GLP-1 (glucagon-like peptide-1)

Table 3
Combination products

Generic Name	Brand Name	Available Dosage Forms	Components
Premixed Combination Insulin Products			
NPH/regular 70/30	Novolin 70/30, Humulin 70/30	U-100 vial, U-100 prefilled pen	70% insulin isophane, 30% human insulin
Lispro 50/50	Humalog Mix 50/50	U-100 vial, U-100 prefilled pen	50% insulin lispro protamine, 50% insulin lispro
Lispro 75/25	Humalog 75/25	U-100 vial, U-100 prefilled pen	75% insulin lispro protamine, 25% insulin lispro
Aspart 70/30	Novolog Mix 70/30	U-100 via, U-100 prefilled pen	70% insulin aspart protamine, 30% insulin aspart
Premixed Insulin/GLP-1 Receptor Antagonist Combination Products			
Degludec/ Liraglutide	Xultophy	3-mL prefilled pen	100 units insulin degludec and 3.6 mg liraglutide per mL
Glargine/ Lixisenatide	Soliqua	3-mL prefilled pen	100 units insulin glargine and 33 µg lixisenatide per mL

Abbreviation: GLP-1, glucagon-like peptide-1.
  Data from Refs.[2,35–40]

receptor antagonist because of its ability to decrease glucose levels effectively, and improved side effect profile compared with increasing the insulin dose.[2] At present 2 combination products are commercially available: insulin glargine plus lixisenatide and insulin degludec plus liraglutide (see **Table 3**).

If clinicians opt to intensify insulin therapy rather than using combination injectable therapy, prandial insulin therapy is typically added to basal insulin. Prandial insulin therapy is most commonly initiated with the largest meal of the day and can be increased to be dosed at other meals if clinically appropriate. Typically, a dose of 4 units or 10% of the basal dose at each meal is given and titrated based on patient response.[2] Multiple prandial products exist and specific information relating to timing with meals is described in **Table 1**.

It may also be possible to convert patients to a regimen consisting of 2 to 3 doses of a premixed combination insulin if cost, resistance to additional injections, or other patient-specific factors necessitate this.[2]

Note that metformin therapy should be continued in patients with T2DM who are receiving combination injectable therapy. Other oral agents, including sulfonylureas and dipeptidyl peptidase-4 inhibitors, are usually not continued because of the risk of adverse effects, including profound hypoglycemia. Occasionally other agents, such as a thiazolidinedione or sodium-glucose cotransporter-2 inhibitors, may be used as part of combination therapy with insulin to improve glycemic control and decrease insulin requirements, although the risks of this approach must be carefully considered.[2]

As patients age or lose functional capacity, simplification of insulin regimens may be warranted. Clinicians should continually reevaluate insulin therapy and individualize regimens as appropriate.[2]

INSULIN THERAPY IN THE INPATIENT SETTING

It is common for hospitalized patients (even those without diabetes mellitus) to experience hyperglycemia caused by the stress response of acute illness. Increased morbidity and mortality are associated with both hypoglycemia and hyperglycemia; therefore, it is paramount to safely achieve target blood glucose concentrations. Insulin is generally the preferred agent to manage hyperglycemia in the inpatient setting and should be started when blood glucose concentrations consistently exceed 180 mg/dL. Once insulin therapy is initiated, the target blood glucose range for most hospitalized patients is 140 to 180 mg/dL, although certain populations may benefit from tighter glycemic control and goals of 110 to 140 mg/dL if these can be achieved safely.[10]

Continuous intravenous (IV) insulin infusions are preferred for critically ill patients experiencing blood glucose levels greater than 180 mg/dL (including patients with diabetic ketoacidosis) because of the ability to easily titrate doses to achieve glycemic targets. Insulin infusion protocols that include frequent blood glucose monitoring, specific titration parameters, and detailed information regarding hypoglycemia prevention and management should be implemented.[11] Subcutaneous basal insulin should be initiated 2 to 4 hours before the IV insulin infusion is discontinued and can be dosed at 60% to 80% of the daily IV insulin infusion rate.[10]

Hospitalized patients with T1DM should receive weight-based basal insulin along with correction-dose insulin and prandial insulin if the patient is able to consume an oral diet.[10]

In non–intensive care unit settings, scheduled insulin therapy is preferred to monotherapy with correction or sliding-scale insulin regimens in patients with diabetes who are experiencing hyperglycemia. Basal insulin or a basal plus bolus correction insulin is recommended by the ADA in non–critically ill patients who are nil by mouth or who have little oral intake. Rapid or short-acting insulin can be administered before meals or every 4 to 6 hours if no meals are administered or in patients who are receiving continuous enteral or parenteral nutrition. Patients with good nutritional intake should receive an insulin regimen consisting of basal, prandial, and correction insulin therapy. If patients are eating well, insulin should be scheduled with mealtimes, with point-of-care blood glucose monitoring performed just before meals. If oral intake is poor, it is safer to administer rapid-acting insulin products immediately after eating.[10] Basal-bolus regimens have shown improved blood glycemic control and fewer treatment failures in surgical patients with T2DM compared with sliding-scale insulin.[12] Monotherapy with sliding-scale insulin should be avoided and, if used, should be used for only short durations.[10] Premixed insulin has been evaluated in hospitalized patients and was associated with an increased risk of hypoglycemia compared with basal-bolus therapy; therefore, it is not preferred.[13] Insulin vials are typically used in the inpatient setting. If insulin pens are used, they must be labeled for single-patient use only. The use of a single insulin pen in multiple patients should be avoided because of the risk of blood-borne infections.[14]

INSULIN DELIVERY DEVICES

Most insulin products are now available in syringe and insulin pen formulations. Product selection should be determined based on a variety of factors, including patient preference, insulin product required, dosing regimen, cost, and ability to administer products correctly. Insulin pens or injection aids may be appropriate in patients with decreased vision or dexterity issues.[15]

Continuous subcutaneous insulin infusions (insulin pumps) offer another option for patients and provide rapid-acting insulin throughout the day. Pumps are considered an appropriate therapy option for patients with T1DM. The use of these devices can be considered for all children and adolescents, especially in children less than 7 years old. The choice of using a pump or managing insulin with multiple daily injections should be made on an individual patient basis.[15]

Another less traditional insulin delivery option is available in a patchlike device that acts to provide a set rate of short-acting basal insulin throughout the day and provides on-demand bolus insulin.[15,16]

Approved in 2014, inhaled insulin (or technosphere insulin) is another option for patients with T1DM and T2DM. One formulation is available and acts as a rapid-acting insulin. No long-acting inhaled insulin products are available on the US market, so patients should be counseled that although inhaled insulin can provide rapid-acting insulin coverage, it cannot replace injections with long-acting insulin. Common adverse reactions unique to inhaled insulin include cough, bronchospasm, decreased pulmonary function, and throat pain or irritation. Before beginning therapy, potential underlying lung disease should be investigated by performing a detailed medical history, physical examination, and spirometry. This medication is not recommended in patients who smoke and it is contraindicated in patients with chronic lung disease (asthma or chronic obstructive lung disease). Lung cancer has also been reported with inhaled insulin and the risks of this must be considered before using this therapy.[17]

Inhaled insulin provided similar A1c reductions to insulin aspart in patients with T1DM, although more patients receiving aspart reached goal A1c levels. The inhaled insulin group had fewer episodes of hypoglycemia and more weight loss, but reported more cough.[18] In addition, a 2015 meta-analysis of technosphere inhaled insulin trials

Table 4	
Insulin storage	
Product	**Opened Room Temperature Storage (d)**
Rapid-acting Insulins	
Novolog	28
Fiasp vial and pen	28
Fiasp cartridges	28
Humalog vial, cartridges, and pens	28
Admelog vial and pen	28
Apidra vial and pen	28
Afrezza	Unopened blister cards + strips: 10 Opened strips: 3
Short-acting Insulins	
Humulin R vials	31
Novolin R vial	42
Novolin R pen	28
Humulin R U-500 pen	28
Humulin R U-500 multiple dose vial	40
Intermediate-acting Insulins	
Humulin N vials	31
Humulin N pen	14
Novolin N vial	42
Novolin N pen	28
Long-acting Insulins	
Tresiba products	56
Levemir products	42
Lantus products	28
Basaglar	28
Toujeo	28
Combination Products	
Novolin 70/30 vial	42
Novolin 70/30 pen	28
Humulin 70/30 vials	31
Humulin 70/30 pen	10
Humalog 50/50 vial	28
Humalog 50/50 pen	10
Humalog 75/25 vial	28
Humalog 75/25 pen	10
Novolog Mix 70/30 vial	28
Novolog Mix 70/30 pen	14
Xultophy	21
Soliqua	14

Data from Refs.[3,4,17,21–24,26–40]

showed lower glycemic efficacy of inhaled insulin versus subcutaneous insulin, but lower risk of severe hypoglycemia and weight gain.[19]

INJECTION TECHNIQUE AND COUNSELING POINTS

Patients and/or caregivers should be counseled on the appropriate administration of insulin. Counseling should include information regarding the importance of rotating injection sites, caring for injection sites to avoid infection, and avoidance of unintended intramuscular (IM) delivery.[2] Insulin can be subcutaneously injected into the abdomen, thigh, buttock, and upper arm. A full discussion of appropriate injection technique is beyond the scope of this article, but the reader is directed to the 2016 new insulin delivery recommendations.[20]

Patients receiving inhaled insulin products should receive education on proper inhaler technique and should be instructed to exhale before use, hold the inhaler level throughout administration, position the inhaler in the mouth, tilt the inhaler toward the chin while keeping head level, inhale deeply, and hold their breath for as long as is comfortable.[17]

In addition to education regarding insulin injection technique, the ADA recommends all patients on insulin therapy receive comprehensive education regarding home blood glucose monitoring, appropriate diet, and the importance of understanding the signs and management of hypoglycemia.[2]

Insulin products require storage consideration because all products should be stored in the refrigerator. After being opened or used for the first time, all insulin products must be discarded within a short time frame (**Table 4**). Counsel patients to adhere to expiration dates to increase efficacy and limit infection risk.

PRESCRIBING CONSIDERATIONS

Insulin requires a delivery device such as syringes or pen needles. Insulin syringes are kept behind the counter in most pharmacies and some states have specific requirements for dispensing of these syringes. Insulin pen needles require a prescription and an International Statistical Classification of Diseases and Related Health Problems, 10th Revision (ICD-10), code on the prescription for dispensing.

Care should be taken to ensure the appropriate pen needle or syringe needle is chosen; 4-mm, 30-gauge pen needles are generally preferred. If syringe needles are used, 6-mm, 30-gauge syringe needles are recommended. Syringe needles are not recommended in very young children (<6 years of age) or in extremely thin adults (body mass index <19 kg/m^2) because of the risk of inadvertent IM injection.[2,20]

SUMMARY

Insulin therapy remains an effective option for treating hyperglycemia in many patients with diabetes. The various insulin products and strategies discussed earlier all have strengths and limitations. Basal and prandial regimens may be appropriate for patients who do not have consistent mealtime schedules, but some basal insulin products are cost-prohibitive for certain patients. Premixed combination insulins may offer a more cost-effective method of providing insulin throughout the day, although less flexibility exists with the dosing of these products because of the inherent nature of the combination product. Inhaled insulin may be an option for patients with no history of lung disease who wish to decrease the number of daily insulin injections. Patient-specific factors must be considered when developing an insulin regimen.

DECLARATION OF CONFLICTING INTERESTS

The author declared no potential conflicts of interests to the research, authorship, and/or publication of this article.

REFERENCES

1. American Diabetes Association. History of diabetes. Available at: http://www.diabetes.org/research-and-practice/student-resources/history-of-diabetes.html. Accessed August 3, 2019.
2. American Diabetes Association. Pharmacologic approaches to glycemic treatment: standards of medical care in diabetes-2019. Diabetes Care 2019; 42(Suppl 1):S90–102.
3. Humulin R U-500 [package insert]. Indianapolis (IN): Eli Lilly and Company; 2018.
4. Humalog [package insert]. Indianapolis (IN): Eli Lilly and Company; 2018.
5. Horvath K, Jeitler K, Berghold A, et al. Long-acting insulin analogues versus NPH insulin (human isophane insulin) for type 2 diabetes mellitus. Cochrane Database Syst Rev 2007;(2):CD005613.
6. Owens DR, Traylor L, Mullins P, et al. Patient-level meta-analysis of efficacy and hypoglycaemia in people with type 2 diabetes initiating insulin glargine 100U/mL or neutral protamine Hagedorn insulin analysed according to concomitant oral antidiabetes therapy. Diabetes Res Clin Pract 2017;124:57–65.
7. Bolli GB, Riddle MC, Bergenstal RM, et al. New insulin glargine 300 U/ml compared with glargine 100 U/ml in insulin-naive people with type 2 diabetes on oral glucose-lowering drugs: a randomized controlled trial (EDITION 3). Diabetes Obes Metab 2015;17(4):386–94.
8. Marso SP, Buse JB. Safety of degludec versus glargine in type 2 diabetes. N Engl J Med 2017;377(20):1995–6.
9. Wysham C, Bhargava A, Chaykin L, et al. Effect of insulin degludec vs insulin glargine U100 on hypoglycemia in patients with type 2 diabetes: the SWITCH 2 randomized clinical trial. JAMA 2017;318(1):45–56.
10. American Diabetes Association. Diabetes care in the hospital: standards of medical care in diabetes-2019. Diabetes Care 2019;42(Suppl 1):S173–81.
11. Jacobi J, Bircher N, Krinsley J, et al. Guidelines for the use of an insulin infusion for the management of hyperglycemia in critically ill patients. Crit Care Med 2012; 40(12):3251–76.
12. Umpierrez GE, Smiley D, Hermayer K, et al. Randomized study comparing a basal-bolus with a basal plus correction insulin regimen for the hospital management of medical and surgical patients with type 2 diabetes: basal plus trial. Diabetes Care 2013;36(8):2169–74.
13. Bellido V, Suarez L, Rodriguez MG, et al. Comparison of basal-bolus and premixed insulin regimens in hospitalized patients with type 2 diabetes. Diabetes Care 2015;38(12):2211–6.
14. U.S. Food and Drug Administration. FDA Drug Safety Communication: FDA requires label warnings to prohibit sharing of multi-dose diabetes pen devices among patients. Available at: https://www.fda.gov/drugs/drug-safety-and-availability/fda-drug-safety-communication-fda-requires-label-warnings-prohibit-sharing-multi-dose-diabetes-pen. Accessed August 3, 2019.
15. American Diabetes Association. Diabetes technology: standards of medical care in diabetes-2019. Diabetes Care 2019;42(Suppl 1):S71–80.

16. Winter A, Lintner M, Knezevich E. V-Go insulin delivery system versus multiple daily insulin injections for patients with uncontrolled type 2 diabetes mellitus. J Diabetes Sci Technol 2015;9(5):1111–6.
17. Afrezza [package insert]. Danbury (CT): MannKind Corporation; 2018.
18. Bode BW, McGill JB, Lorber DL, et al. Inhaled technosphere insulin compared with injected prandial insulin in type 1 diabetes: a randomized 24-Week trial. Diabetes Care 2015;38(12):2266–73.
19. Pittas AG, Westcott GP, Balk EM. Efficacy, safety, and patient acceptability of Technosphere inhaled insulin for people with diabetes: a systematic review and meta-analysis. Lancet Diabetes Endocrinol 2015;3(11):886–94.
20. Frid AH, Kreugel G, Grassi G, et al. New insulin delivery recommendations. Mayo Clin Proc 2016;91(9):1231–55.
21. Admelog [package insert]. Bridgewater (NJ): Sanofi-Aventis U.S. LLC; 2018.
22. Apidra [package insert]. Bridgewater (NJ): Sanofi-Aventis U.S. LLC; 2018.
23. Fiasp [package insert]. Plainsboro (NJ): Novo Nordisk Inc.; 2018.
24. Novolog [package insert]. Plainsboro (NJ): Novo Nordisk; 2019.
25. Admelog [package insert]. In. Bridgewater (NJ): Sanofi-Aventis U.S. LLC; 2018.
26. Humulin R [package insert]. Indianapolis (IN): Eli Lilly and Company; 2018.
27. Novolin R [package insert]. Plainsboro (NJ): Novo Nordisk Inc; 2018.
28. Humulin N [package insert]. Indianapolis (IN): Eli Lilly and Company; 2018.
29. Novolin N [package insert]. Plainsboro (NJ): Novo Nordisk Inc; 2018.
30. Tresiba [package insert]. Plainsboro (NJ): Novo Nordisk Inc.; 2018.
31. Levemir [package insert]. Plainsboro (NJ): Novo Nordisk Inc.; 2019.
32. Lantus [package insert]. Bridgewater (NJ): Sanofi-Aventis; 2019.
33. Basaglar [package insert]. Ridgefield (CT): Eli Lilly and Company; 2018.
34. Toujeo [package insert]. Bridgewater (NJ): Sanofi-Aventis; 2019.
35. Humalog Mix 50/50 [package insert]. Indianapolis, IN: Eli Lilly and Company; 2018.
36. Humalog Mix 75/25 [package insert]. Indianapolis (IN): Eli Lilly and Company; 2018.
37. Novolin 70/30 [package insert]. Plainsboro (NJ): Novo Nordisk Inc; 2018.
38. Humulin 70/30 [package insert]. Indianapolis (IN): Eli Lilly and Company; 2018.
39. Xultophy [package insert]. Plainsboro (NJ): Novo Nordisk Inc.; 2019.
40. Soliqua [package insert]. Bridgewater, NJ: Sanofi-Aventis U.S. LLC; 2019.

Managing Diabetes in the Digital Age

Joy A. Dugan, DHSc, MPH, PA-C[a],*, Sumera Ahmed, MD, BC-ADM[b],
Margarita Vincent, MPH(c), PA-S[a], Rosalyn Perry, MPH(c), PA-S[a],
Clipper F. Young, PharmD, MPH, CDE, BC-ADM, BCGP[b]

KEYWORDS

- Diabetic technology • Insulin pump • Continuous glucose meter
- Patient-generated data

KEY POINTS

- Effective technology includes the following components: (1) communication, (2) patient-generated health data, (3) education, and (4) feedback.
- Continuous glucose monitors offer real-time glucose levels and reports on glucose trends that is missed by either a fingerstick glucose or a hemoglobin A_{1C}.
- Insulin pumps offer a more physiologic option to managing diabetes; decreasing hypoglycemic episodes and glucose variability.
- Although not FDA regulated, phone applications and social media platforms are useful for patients needing psychosocial support.

INTRODUCTION

The joint position statement of the American Diabetes Association (ADA), American Association of Diabetes Educators, and the Academy of Nutrition and Dietetics recommends that patients receive diabetes self-management education (DSME) and support services at diagnosis, annually, when complications/comorbidities occur, and during transitions of care (eg, hospitalization, pregnancy).[1] In 2019, for the first time, the 2019 ADA Standards of Medical Care in Diabetes included an article on diabetes technology.[2] The ADA defines diabetes technology as "hardware, devices, and software that people with diabetes use to help manage blood glucose levels, stave off diabetes complications, reduce the burden of living with diabetes and improve the quality of life."[2]

---

[a] Joint MSPAS/MPH Program, Touro University California, 1310 Johnson Lane, Vallejo, CA 94592, USA; [b] College of Osteopathic Medicine, Touro University California, 1310 Johnson Lane, Vallejo, CA 94592, USA
* Corresponding author.
E-mail address: Joy.dugan@tu.edu

Physician Assist Clin 5 (2020) 177–190
https://doi.org/10.1016/j.cpha.2019.12.003
2405-7991/20/© 2020 Elsevier Inc. All rights reserved.
physicianassistant.theclinics.com

KEY COMPONENTS OF TECHNOLOGY FOR DIABETES SELF-MANAGEMENT EDUCATION

The most effective technology includes the following components for hemoglobin (Hb) A_{1c} management[3]:

- Communication
- Patient-generated health data
- Education
- Feedback

The most effective technology allows patients to access their diabetes health care team with patient-specific health data and customized feedback via two-way communication. Opportunities that promote shared decision making between patients and providers are necessary for positive diabetes outcomes.[3]

EFFECT ON DIABETES OUTCOMES

In a 2017 meta-analysis, patient satisfaction, self-efficacy, blood pressure, and weight management were all improved with the use of technology-enhanced DSME.[3] Diabetes distress, defined as the "unique, often hidden burdens and worries that are part of a patient experience when managing a severe, demanding chronic disease like diabetes," also improves when technology is integrated into DSME.[4] Diabetes self-management programs that integrate technology have shown to improve HbA_{1c} up to 0.8%.

CONTINUOUS GLUCOSE MONITORS
Introduction to Continuous Glucose Monitors

Continuous glucose monitors (CGMs) have gained popularity in diabetes management because they bridge the inherent gaps in the other means of assessing glycemic control. Other forms of testing including fingerstick glucose testing and HbA_{1c} do not capture the daily glycemic fluctuations and trends.[2] The first CGM, developed in 1999, was a retrospective monitor, allowing the user to view trends of their interstitial fluid glucose levels.[2,5,6] Now, CGMs offer real-time glucose monitoring and alert the user when glucose levels are either lower or higher than the programmed range.[7] The four companies that manufacture CGMs in the United States are compared in **Table 1**. There is only one implantable CGM, Eversense, inserted in-office and worn in the arm for up to 90 days.[8,9]

Several clinical trials comparing CGM with self-management blood glucose in type 1 (T1DM) and type 2 (T2DM) diabetes showed a statistically significant decrease in HbA_{1c} from baseline and shortened duration of hypoglycemia episodes in the CGM users.[10–15] Improved HbA_{1c} values are obtained in CGM users regardless of insulin delivery methods.[16] Proven via various clinical trials and systematic reviews, CGMs are safe and effective for T1DM and T2DM.[17] Patients with T1DM who use CGMs have also reported improved quality of life in relation to hypoglycemia awareness and diabetes distress.[18]

Limitations of Continuous Glucose Monitors

Before 2017, it was necessary for users to recalibrate CGMs every 12 hours. This required the user to check a fingerstick blood glucose and enter that value into an insulin pump that paired with the device.[19] With the new sensor technology, some CGM devices eliminated the need for the user to use fingerstick blood glucose readings to ensure the accuracy of the sensor.[19,20] Even though the number of CGM users is

Table 1
Comparison of common continuous glucose monitors

	Dexcom G6[56]	Freestyle Libre[57]	Medtronic Guardian[58]	Eversense[9]
Sensor wear	10 d	14 d	7 d	3 mo
Sensor location	Stomach; buttock option if 2–17 y/o	Back of upper arm	Back of upper arm or stomach	Back of upper arm
Warm-up period	2 h	1 h	2 h	10 min
Reading frequency	Every 5 min	Every min	Every 5 min	Every 5 min
Fingerstick required	No[a,b] Factory calibrated	No[a] Factory calibrated	Twice/day for calibration	Twice/day for calibration
Coverage	Medicare, most commercial plans	Medicare, most commercial plans	Most commercial plans, but not Medicare	Plan specific
Age group	≥2 year old	≥18 year old	14–75 year old	≥18 year old
Device receivers and reader	Dexcom receiver or smart device	Libre Receiver	Smart device (excludes Android)	Smart device
Shareable glucose data	Directly up to 5 people	Indirectly via link or pdf of data upload	Directly up to 5 people	Directly up to 5 people
Water-resistant	Yes[c]	Yes[c]	Yes[d]	Yes[c]

Chart Author: Amanda Flohr, MSPAS, MPH, PA-C.
[a] Meter may prompt manual calibration with fingerstick if there is an error.
[b] First two calibrations occur within 2 hours after connecting new sensor and within 6 hours after first calibration; then continue with subsequent calibrations.
[c] Up to 3.2 feet (1 m) for 30 minutes.
[d] Up to 8 feet (2.4 m) for 30 minutes.
Data from Refs.[9,56–58]

increasing, there are still perceived barriers by patients to incorporate the technology, including user-perceived accuracy of self-management blood glucose over CGM, the cost, and the discomfort when wearing the device.[21] Addressing these concerns requires further patient education.[19]

Interpreting Continuous Glucose Monitor Data

The standardized CGM report consists of two components: glucose patterns summary with core CGM metrics, and ambulatory glucose profile with a visual display of daily glucose levels. The core CGM metrics include average glucose, glucose management index (an estimate HbA$_{1c}$ from CGM data), time in range, time in hypoglycemia, time in hyperglycemia, and glucose variability quantifying blood glucose control.[16]

The time in range commonly guides diabetes management with 70 to 180 mg/dL as the default range,[22] summarizing the portion/percentage of CGM data falls within this range during a measurement period. A higher percentage for time in range indicates higher degree of blood glucose control. However, readings falling outside of the desired blood glucose range (ie, time in hypoglycemia and time in hyperglycemia) should be minimized with continuous refinements on diabetes management approaches.

An ambulatory glucose profile report is a personalized feedback tool reflecting glycemic patterns throughout the day (**Fig. 1**). It can identify the specific hours during the day when the patient experienced out-of-range blood glucose levels whether hypoglycemic or hyperglycemic. The goal is to keep the blood sugar within the target range as much as possible. This is accomplished by flattening and narrowing the shaded (target) area.

Future Development of Continuous Glucose Monitors

More devices are currently in research including a wearable eye contact lens, which can perform CGM using biosensors to measure glucose levels in tears, and a subcutaneous implant that will operate for a few days and is replaced by the patient.[23,24]

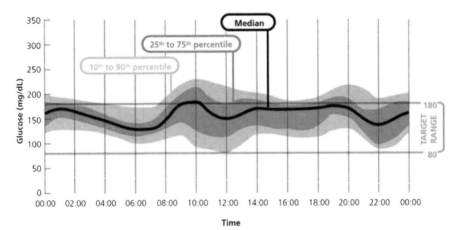

Fig. 1. Sample CGM data. The *solid line* represents the median. The *darkly shaded region* around the *solid line* is the interquartile range (data between the 25th and 75th percentiles), representing glucose variability. The *two horizontal lines* indicate the target range (eg, 70 and 180 mg/dL).

INSULIN PUMPS
History of Insulin Pumps

In 1963, the first insulin pump was invented by Dr Arnold Kadish for research use and was designed as a large backpack.[25] Current insulin pumps are comparable in size to a smartphone. The advent of real-time CGM has allowed the development of sensor-augmented pump (SAP), consisting of a CGM plus an insulin pump. With SAP, patients can better manage glucose levels through increased glucose monitoring, automated insulin suspension, and a bolus calculator feature.[26] However, limitations of SAPs include the need to manually modify basal rates and the inability to automatically deliver bolus or correction insulin.[26] The newest technology currently on the market includes a hybrid closed-loop (HCL) insulin delivery system that uses advanced algorithms to allow automatic adjustments to basal insulin delivery, which overcomes the deficiencies in SAPs.[27]

How Does an Insulin Pump Work?

An insulin pump is a computerized, battery-operated device that allows continuous subcutaneous delivery of insulin through an infusion set or a patch (**Figs. 2** and **3**). There is a basic vocabulary associated with insulin pumps (**Box 1**). The device is worn outside the body and attempts to mimic normal pancreas action by releasing insulin via a programmed basal and bolus insulin delivery (**Table 2**).

Pumps can use any rapid-acting insulin, which is stored inside a cartridge. Insulin is delivered from the cartridge through a flexible tubing that ends in a tiny needle or flexible plastic subcutaneous cannula. The needle or cannula is held in place by an infusion set with an adhesive patch adhering to the skin (**Table 3**).

Hybrid Closed-Loop Insulin Pumps

The HCL algorithms require glucose measurements from real-time CGM while patients must still manually adjust bolus insulin.[28] The HCL systems show the greatest improvements in glucose control, increased time spent in target glucose range, decreased HbA$_{1c}$ levels, reduction of hypoglycemic and diabetic ketoacidosis events, and reduced

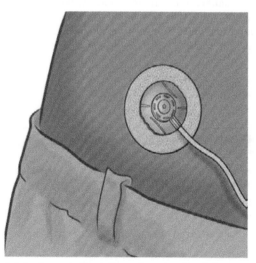

Fig. 2. Illustration of infusion set. Depiction of an insulin delivery set-up for an insulin pump. (*Courtesy of* A. Peters, MD, Los Angeles, CA.)

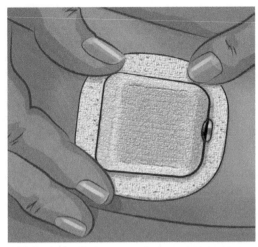

Fig. 3. Illustration of the Omnipod. (*Courtesy of* A. Peters, MD, Los Angeles, CA.)

bolus delivery in T1DM patients, both children and adults.[19,29,30] Another advancement includes technology to control basal rate using an algorithm to predict low blood glucose levels based on CGM trends.[19] This feature allows the pump to cease insulin delivery before glucose levels reach predetermined low levels.[19] At present, there are few studies on HCL systems and effects on T2DM.

Current Challenges with Insulin Pumps

The exceptional outcomes and benefits achieved with HCL therapy have demonstrated extensive progress toward creating an entirely closed-loop system. However, there are existing limitations and challenges (**Table 4**). At this time, HCL therapy still requires patients to manually calculate and enter the amount of carbohydrates for meals and thus is still not an exclusively closed-loop system.[28] A dangerous and potential complication includes infusion set failure, which may lead to rapid diabetic ketoacidosis.[29] Patients should be counseled to follow manufacturer recommendations for set changes to optimize diabetes management.

Factors that may negatively impact or hinder access to insulin pump therapy include[31,32]

- Lower socioeconomic status
- Language barriers

Box 1
Continuous glucose monitors and insulin pump terminology

- Basal rate: constant supply of insulin delivered automatically at a personalized, preset rate around the clock mimicking pancreatic basal secretion. Concept is to simulate the pancreas.

- Bolus: additional insulin doses delivered as needed either around mealtime for carbohydrate coverage or to correct high blood glucose.

- Daily totals: total insulin delivered (basal + bolus) in the last 24-hour period.

- Suspend: insulin delivery (both basal + bolus) is stopped.

- "Sets" (or infusion set): the attachment from the insulin pump to the patient's body.

Table 2
Advantages and disadvantages of insulin pump therapy

Advantages of Insulin Pump Therapy	Potential Disadvantages of Insulin Pump Therapy
More physiologic and precise insulin delivery and absorption More convenient and discrete injections Reduces risk of hypoglycemia and severe hypoglycemia Improves HbA$_{1c}$ level Reduces glycemic variability Flexible lifestyle	Risk of skin reactions/infections Possible infusion set malfunction can potentiate diabetic ketoacidosis Device attached to body Cost

Data from Grunberger G, Abelseth J, Bailey T, Bode B, Handelsman Y, Hellman R, Jovanovic L... et al. Consensus Statement by the American Association of Clinical Endocrinologists/American College of Endocrinology Insulin Pump Management Task Force. *Endocrine Practice*, 2014; 20(4):463-439. Retrieved from https://www.aace.com/disease-state-resources/diabetes/position-and-consensus-statements/consensus-statement-american.

Table 3
Insulin pump types

Pump Type	Tandem t:slimX2[59]	Medtronic: MiniMed 630G and MiniMed 670G[60] (500 series are older versions)	Insulet Omnipod[61] (See Fig. 3)
Claim to fame	Almost closed-loop system and only pump with rechargeable battery	Almost closed-loop system	Only tubeless or "patch" pump available in the United States
Hypoglycemia reduction	Basal-IQ technology that predicts glucose levels 30 min ahead (based on in-built algorithm) and suspends insulin if they are expected to drop lower than 80 mg/dL This feature helps reduce the frequency and duration of hypoglycemia Once glucose level rises, system resumes insulin delivery	SmartGuard technology pauses insulin delivery for up to 2 h if the sensor glucose values go lower than a preset level This helps prevent severe hypoglycemia In auto mode, pump automatically adjusts basal based on CGM readings and predictive algorithms	Omnipod has partnered with Dexcom CGM Although there are no integrated algorithms to prevent hypoglycemia, the Omnipod has the ability to share information with up to 12 friends or family members on smartphone
Hardware compatibility	T:slimX2 integrates with Dexcom G6 CGM Does not link to any glucometer	Integrates with Medtronic Guardian Connect CGM and Contour Next Link 2.4 m	The Contour Next One blood glucose meter communicates with Omnipod DASH system and Dexcom G5/6 CGM
Water exposure	Watertight to 3 feet for up to 30 min	Water resistant to 12 feet for 24 h	Pod is waterproof for up to 25 feet for 60 min

Data from Refs.[59–61]

Table 4 Considerations for insulin pump candidates	
Patients Who Will Not Do Well with Pump Therapy	**Recommended Insulin Pump Candidate**
Do not check fingerstick blood glucose at least 4 times a day	T1DM
	Glycemic goal difficult to achieve despite MDI
Do not do MDI	Extreme insulin sensitivity (labile diabetes)
Unable to do carbohydrate counting	Frequent severe hypoglycemia
Lack motivation for better glucose control	Hypoglycemia unawareness
Unstable mental health	High glycemic variability
Extremely conscious about device on body	Variable work/activity schedules
Unrealistic expectations of pump therapy with misbelief that it will eliminate glucose monitoring	Pregnancy in T1DM
	Selected T2DM patients with high glycemic variability, suboptimal control despite maximal regimen of MDI

Abbreviation: MDI, multiple daily injections.
Data from Grunberger G, Abelseth J, Bailey T, Bode B, et al. Consensus Statement by the American Association of Clinical Endocrinologists/American College of Endocrinology Insulin Pump Management Task Force. *Endocr Pract.* 2014 May;20(5):463-89 Retrieved from https://www.aace.com/disease-state-resources/diabetes/position-and-consensus-statements/consensus-statement-american

- Preferences of the patient regarding device appearance
- Interference with physical activities
- Provider implicit bias

An additional challenge is that many providers lack sufficient knowledge or education on how to use pump devices.[32]

Do-It-Yourself Artificial Pancreas

Technology-savvy individuals have created do-it-yourself closed-loop systems. The Open Artificial Pancreas System project and Loop app template provide instructions on how to construct automated closed-loop systems using currently available technologies.[33–35] However, this requires users to gain unauthorized access or "hack" insulin pumps and CGMs that have not been Food and Drug Administration (FDA)-approved for this type of use. Tidepool is a nonprofit organization for diabetes technology studying the Loop app and its use in self-management. If the FDA approves this smartphone app in the future, individuals will be able to pair their insulin pump and CGM for customized blood glucose management.

PATIENT-GENERATED HEALTH DATA

Patient-generated health data (PGHD) can include fitness trackers, food logs, and CGM systems. Ideally, providers should be able to review and provide feedback on this information. However, many health care teams may not be prepared to analyze PGHD.[3] Being able to incorporate PGHD into the medical record would provide a comprehensive analysis of patient daily activity, its effect on various chronic diseases, and provide insight into the patient's habits allowing the practitioner to guide management.[36] A systematic review of 67 randomized controlled trials showed a significant reduction with the incorporation of PGHD in HbA_{1c} numbers, blood pressure, total cholesterol, and triglycerides in comparison with standard care.[37] PGHD-guided treatment has the most benefit to those patients who continuously engage in monitoring health data.[38,39]

Phone Applications

Mobile phone apps are being used in various ways to assist in DSME by providing insight into lifestyle management factors, such as diet, exercise, and medication adherence through reminders. Phone apps that provide community support reduce HbA$_{1c}$ by as much as 0.5% especially among those with T2DM.[40–43] Although numerous health-themed phone apps are available, there is no regulatory body monitoring the information provided.[44] The FDA only regulates apps that are being used as treatment, such as apps that interface with an insulin pump or CGM. **Table 5** shows several recommended phone apps.[45]

Social Media

A growing number of individuals use the Internet, including social media sites, for health care information.[46] Patients with diabetes who use diabetes-specific social media sites may wish to share or seek advice regarding diabetes care and/or lifestyle changes to better cope with their daily management.[47] Various research studies have shown that social networking sites are able to improve glycemic control, improve knowledge of disease, and increase social support.[47–49]

Cybersecurity

As diabetes technologies have significantly advanced over recent years, connection of such devices through wireless communication has also increased.[6] The use of wireless connection increases the risk of unauthorized third parties gaining access to

Table 5
Phone applications and associated features

Application	Glucose Buddy	MySugr Diabetes Logbook	Diabetes Connect	Sugar Sense	One Drop	Diabetes and Blood Glucose Tracker (Apple)	Diabetes and Diet Tracker (Android)	BG Monitor Diabetes
Cost	Free	$2.99/mo	$1.99/mo	Free	$39.95/mo	$9/mo	$9/mo	Free
Healthy eating	Yes	Yes	Yes	Yes	Yes	Yes	Yes	No
Being active	Yes	No	Yes	Yes	Yes	Yes	Yes	No
Monitoring	Yes	Yes	Yes	Yes	Yes	No	No	Yes
Taking medications	Yes	Yes	Yes	Yes	Yes	Yes	Yes	Yes
Reducing risks	No	Yes	No	Yes	No	Yes	Yes	No
Problem solving	No	Yes	Yes	No	Yes	Yes	Yes	Yes
Healthy coping	Yes	No	No	No	Yes	Yes	Yes	No
Syncs with meters	No	No	No	No	Yes	Yes	Yes	No
Community support	Yes	Yes	Yes	No	Yes	Yes	Yes	No

diabetes devices.[50] As such, potential for breaches of personal health information data should be considered with new technologies.[3,51–53] It is crucial to note that a breach in security could alter the commands and information flowing between diabetes devices.[6,51,52] There is an increased risk of compromising the successful and safe functioning of such devices.[6,52,54] A compromised device can result in decreased control of blood glucose and an undesirable health complication for the user.[6,52]

Recognizing the inherent risks of security breaches, the Diabetes Technology Society founded the Diabetes Technology Society Cybersecurity Standard for Connected Diabetes Devices project.[51,54,55] The project aims to preserve device function, protect confidential patient information, and prevent unauthorized modification or disclosure from the potential negative health effects and outcomes of compromised device security.[6,50,55] Assurance and performance requirements were also developed, which assists independent entities in conducting assessments on connected diabetes device.[51]

SUMMARY

Technology in DSME can improve the quality of life and decrease stress levels of individuals living with diabetes.[3] In the 100 years since the discovery of insulin, multiple advances in diabetes technology continue to improve the lives of individuals with diabetes. When helping patients decide about CGMs and insulin pumps, consider referring patients to http://www.diabeteswise.org, a resource for patients to help them make the right lifestyle choice about diabetes technology. The Web site is sponsored by an initiative by people with diabetes and Stanford University. Practitioners should be familiar with the technological advances in diabetes to help educate patients in opportunities for improving control and quality of life.

DISCLOSURES

We have no disclosures.

REFERENCES

1. Powers MA, Bardsley J, Cypress M, et al. Diabetes self-management education and support in type 2 diabetes: a joint position statement of the American Diabetes Association, the American Association of Diabetes Educators, and the Academy of Nutrition and Dietetics. Diabetes Educ 2015;41(4):417–30.
2. American Diabetes Association. Diabetes technology: standards of medical care in diabetes—2019. Diabetes Care 2019;42(Supplement 1):S71–80.
3. Greenwood DA, Gee PM, Fatkin KJ, et al. A systematic review of reviews evaluating technology-enabled diabetes self-management education and support. J Diabetes Sci Technol 2017;11(5):1015–27.
4. Fisher L, Hessler DM, Polonsky WH, et al. When is diabetes distress clinically meaningful? Diabetes Care 2012;35(2):259–64.
5. Weaver K, Hirsch IB. The hybrid closed-loop system: evolution and practical applications. Diabetes Technol Ther 2018;20(S2):S216–23.
6. Klonoff DC. Cybersecurity for connected diabetes devices. J Diabetes Sci Technol 2015;9(5):1143–7.
7. Heinermann L, Stuhr A, Brown A, et al. Self-measurement of blood glucose and continuous glucose monitoring: is there only one future? Eur Endocrinol 2018; 14(2):24–9.

8. Food & Drug Administration. Eversense CGM sensor insertion and removal instruction. 2017. Available at: https://www.fda.gov/media/112159/download. Accessed July 24, 2019.

9. Senseonics. Eversense: user guide: a guide for using the Eversense continuous glucose monitoring system. 2018. Available at: https://www.eversensediabetes.com/wp-content/uploads/2018/08/LBL-1602-01-001-Rev-D_Eversense-User-Guide_mgdL_R1-2.pdf. Accessed January 15, 2020.

10. Juvenile Diabetes Research Foundation Continuous Glucose Monitoring Study Group, Tamborlane WV, Beck RW, Bode BW, et al. Continuous glucose monitoring and intensive treatment of type 1 diabetes. N Engl J Med 2008;359(14):1464–76.

11. Beck RW, Riddlesworth T, Ruedy K, et al. Effect of continuous glucose monitoring on glycemic control in adults with type 1 diabetes using insulin injections: the DIAMOND randomized clinical trial. JAMA 2017;317(4):371–8.

12. Beck RW, Riddlesworth TD, Ruedy K, et al. Continuous glucose monitoring versus usual care in patients with type 2 diabetes receiving multiple daily insulin injections: a randomized trial continuous glucose monitoring in patients with type 2 diabetes. Ann Intern Med 2017;167(6):365–74.

13. Ruedy KJ, Parkin CG, Riddlesworth TD, et al, DIAMOND Study Group. Continuous glucose monitoring in older adults with type 1 and type 2 diabetes using multiple daily injections of insulin: results from the DIAMOND trial. J Diabetes Sci Technol 2017;11(6):1138–46.

14. Vigersky R, Shrivastav M. Role of continuous glucose monitoring for type 2 in diabetes management and research. J Diabetes Complications 2017;31(1):280–7.

15. Ólafsdóttir AF, Polonsky W, Bolinder J, et al. A randomized clinical trial of the effect of continuous glucose monitoring on nocturnal hypoglycemia, daytime hypoglycemia, glycemic variability, and hypoglycemia confidence in persons with type 1 diabetes treated with multiple daily insulin injections (GOLD-3). Diabetes Technol Ther 2018;20(4):274–84.

16. Fonseca VA, Grunberger G, Anhalt H, et al. Continuous glucose monitoring: a consensus conference of the American Association of Clinical Endocrinologists and American College of Endocrinology. Endocr Pract 2016;22(8):1008–21.

17. Rodbard D. Continuous glucose monitoring: a review of recent studies demonstrating improved glycemic outcomes. Diabetes Technol Ther 2017;19(S3):S25–37.

18. Polonsky WH, Hessler D, Ruedy KJ, et al, DIAMOND Study Group. The impact of continuous glucose monitoring on markers of quality of life in adults with type 1 diabetes: further findings from the DIAMOND randomized clinical trial. Diabetes Care 2017;40(6):736–41.

19. Forlenza G, Kushner T, Messer L, et al. Factory-calibrated continuous glucose monitoring: how and why it works, and the dangers of reuse beyond approved duration of wear. Diabetes Technol Ther 2019;21(4):222–9.

20. Hoss U, Budiman ES. Factory-calibrated continuous glucose sensors: the science behind the technology. Diabetes Technol Ther 2017;19(S2):S44–50.

21. Engler R, Routh TL, Lucisano JY. Adoption barriers for continuous glucose monitoring and their potential reduction with a fully implanted system: results from patient preference surveys. Clin Diabetes 2018;36(1):50–8.

22. Hirsch IB, Battelino T, Peters AL, et al. Role of continuous glucose monitoring in diabetes treatment. Arlington (VA): American Diabetes Association; 2018.

23. Chen C, Zhao XL, Li ZH, et al. Current and emerging technology for continuous glucose monitoring. Sensors (Basel) 2017;17(1):182.

24. Elsherif M, Hassan MU, Yetisen AK, et al. Wearable contact lens biosensors for continuous glucose monitoring using smartphones. ACS Nano 2018;12(6): 5452–62.

25. Ghazanfar H, Rizvi SW, Khurram A, et al. Impact of insulin pump on quality of life of diabetic patients. Indian J Endocrinol Metab 2016;20(4):506–11.

26. Steineck I, Ranjan A, Nørgaard K, et al. Sensor-augmented insulin pumps and hypoglycemia prevention in type 1 diabetes. J Diabetes Sci Technol 2016; 11(1):50–8.

27. Garg SK, Weinzimer SA, Tamborlane WV, et al. Glucose outcomes with the in-home use of a hybrid closed-loop insulin delivery system in adolescents and adults with type 1 diabetes. Diabetes Technol Ther 2017;19(3):155–63.

28. McAuley SA, de Bock MI, Sundararajan V, et al. Effect of 6 months of hybrid closed-loop insulin delivery in adults with type 1 diabetes: a randomised controlled trial protocol. BMJ Open 2018;8(6):e020274.

29. Tauschmann M, Thabit H, Bally L, et al. Closed-loop insulin delivery in suboptimally controlled type 1 diabetes: a multicentre, 12-week randomised trial [published correction appears in Lancet. 2018;392(10155):1310]. Lancet 2018; 392(10155):1321–9.

30. Tauschmann M, Allen JM, Wilinska ME, et al. Day-and-night hybrid closed-loop insulin delivery in adolescents with type 1 diabetes: a free-living, randomized clinical trial. Diabetes Care 2015;39(7):1168–74.

31. Tanenbaum ML, Hanes SJ, Miller KM, et al. Diabetes device use in adults with type 1 diabetes: barriers to uptake and potential intervention targets. Diabetes Care 2016;40(2):181–7.

32. Tanenbaum ML, Adams RN, Hanes SJ, et al. Optimal use of diabetes devices: clinician perspectives on barriers and adherence to device use. J Diabetes Sci Technol 2017;11(3):484–92.

33. Kowalski A. Taking do-it-yourself artificial pancreas systems mainstream. JDRF. 10/18/17 Available at: https://www.jdrf.org/blog/2017/10/18/taking-artificial-pancreas-systems-mainstream/. Accessed May 8, 2019.

34. LoopDocs. Loop. [online]. 2019. Available at: https://loopkit.github.io/loopdocs/?_ga=2.142178866.1437506049.1557330021-976144178.1557330021#introduction. Accessed May 8, 2019.

35. Openaps.org. What is #OpenAPS? – OpenAPS.org. 2019. Available at: https://openaps.org/what-is-openaps/. Accessed 8 May 2019.

36. Cohen DJ, Keller SR, Hayes GR, et al. Integrating patient-generated health data into clinical care settings or clinical decision-making: lessons learned from project HealthDesign. JMIR Hum Factors 2016;3(2):e26.

37. Or CK, Tao D. Does the use of consumer health information technology improve outcomes in the patient self-management of diabetes? A meta-analysis and narrative review of randomized controlled trials. Int J Med Inform 2014;83(5): 320–9.

38. Garabedian LF, Ross-Degnan D, Wharam JF. Mobile phone and smartphone technologies for diabetes care and self-management. Curr Diab Rep 2015; 15(12):109.

39. Park YR, Lee Y, Kim JY, et al. Managing patient-generated health data through mobile personal health records: analysis of usage data. JMIR Mhealth Uhealth 2018;6(4):e89.

40. El-Gayar O, Timsina P, Nawar N, et al. Mobile applications for diabetes self-management: status and potential. J Diabetes Sci Technol 2013;7(1):247–62.

41. Cui M, Wu X, Mao J, et al. Type 2 diabetes self-management via smartphone applications: a systematic review and meta-analysis. PLoS One 2016;11(11): e0166718.

42. Hou C, Carter B, Hewitt J, et al. Do mobile phone applications improve glycemic control (HbA1c) in the self-management of diabetes? A systematic review, meta-analysis, and GRADE of 14 randomized trials. Diabetes Care 2016;39(11): 2089–95.

43. Wu Y, Yao X, Vespasiani G, et al. Mobile app-based interventions to support diabetes self-management: a systematic review of randomized controlled trials to identify functions associated with glycemic efficacy. JMIR Mhealth Uhealth 2017;5(3):e35.

44. Anderson K, Burford O, Emmerton L. Mobile health apps to facilitate self-care: a qualitative study of user experiences. PLoS One 2016;11(5):e0156164.

45. Kerr D. Smartphone apps for diabetes management. Diabetes forecast. 2017. Available at: http://www.diabetesforecast.org/2017/mar-apr/diabetes-applications. html. Accessed May 3, 2019.

46. Pew Research Center. Internet user demographics. 2018. Available at: www. pewinternet.org/data-trend/internet-use/latest-stats/. Accessed January 15, 2020.

47. Nelakurthi AR, Pinto AM, Cook CB, et al. Should patients with diabetes be encouraged to integrate social media into their care plan? Future Sci OA 2018;4(7): FSO323.

48. Toma T, Athanasiou T, Harling L, et al. Online social networking services in the management of patients with diabetes mellitus: systematic review and meta-analysis of randomised controlled trials. Diabetes Res Clin Pract 2014;106(2): 200–11.

49. Gabarron E, Årsand E, Wynn R. Social media use in interventions for diabetes: rapid evidence-based review. J Med Internet Res 2018;20(8):e10303.

50. Out DJ, Tettero O. Assessing the security of connected diabetes devices. J Diabetes Sci Technol 2017;11(2):203–6.

51. Diabetestechnology.org. Diabetes Technology Society. 2019. Available at: https:// www.diabetestechnology.org/dtsec.shtml?ver=5. Accessed May 3, 2019.

52. Khera M. Think like a hacker. J Diabetes Sci Technol 2017;11(2):207–12.

53. Thiel S, Mitchell J, Williams J. Coordination or collision? The intersection of diabetes care, cybersecurity, and cloud-based computing. J Diabetes Sci Technol 2016;11(2):195–7.

54. Sackner-Bernstein J. Design of hack-resistant diabetes devices and disclosure of their cyber safety. J Diabetes Sci Technol 2017;11(2):198–202.

55. Klonoff DC, Kleidermacher DN. Now is the time for a cybersecurity standard for connected diabetes devices. J Diabetes Sci Technol 2016;10(3):623–6.

56. Dexcom. Dexcom G6 continuous glucose monitoring system: User guide. 2018. Available at: https://s3-us-west-2.amazonaws.com/dexcompdf/G6-CGM-Users-Guide.pdf?_ga=2.254658638.730099590.1540359512-885951046.1539387542&_ gac=1.262590846.1540364533.Cj0KCQjwsMDeBRDMARIsAKrOP7GL5Y2Jqlams lcREqZwzSmL4Gfa73aHoJBiaLX9qacMGizEUyG-wKkaAsDIEALw_wcB. Accessed January 15, 2020.

57. Abbott. FreeStyle libre 14 day flash glucose monitoring system: user's manual. 2018. Available at: https://freestyleserver.com/Payloads/IFU/2018/ART39764-001_rev-A-Web.pdf. Accessed January 15, 2020.

58. Medtronic. Guardian T connect CGM: system user guide. 2018. Available at: https:// www.medtronicdiabetes.com/sites/default/files/library/download-library/user-gui

des/GuardianT%20Connect%20CGM%20System%20User%20Guide.PDF. Accessed July 30, 2019.

59. T:slim X2 insulin pump. 2019. Available at: https://www.tandemdiabetes.com/products/t-slim-x2-insulin-pump. Accessed July 29, 2019.

60. Medtronic insulin pump therapy. 2019. Available at: https://www.medtronicdiabetes.com/treatments/insulin-pump-therapy. Accessed July 30, 2019.

61. Omnipod dash system. 2019. Available at: https://www.myomnipod.com/DASH. Accessed July 30, 2019.

When Crisis Strikes
The Acute Complications of Diabetes

Harvey A. Feldman, MD

KEYWORDS

- Diabetic ketoacidosis • Hyperosmolar hyperglycemic state • Hypoglycemia
- Hypoglycemia unawareness • Hypoglycemia-associated autonomic failure

KEY POINTS

- Diabetic ketoacidosis (DKA) comprises hyperglycemia, ketosis, and metabolic acidosis. Blood glucose is usually greater than 250 mg/dL, but may be "euglycemic" under certain circumstances, including the use of the sodium glucose cotransporter-2 inhibitors.
- Hyperosmolar hyperglycemic state (HHS) comprises severe hyperglycemia, greater than 600 mg/dL, accompanied by severe dehydration, but without ketosis or metabolic acidosis.
- Both DKA and HHS are life threatening and require emergent restoration of circulating blood volume, correction of hyperglycemia, and electrolyte imbalance as well as identification and treatment of precipitating factors.
- Hypoglycemia in diabetes is due to excess insulin or insulin secretagogues combined with decreased secretion of glucagon and hypoglycemia-associated autonomic failure (HAAF). In turn, hypoglycemic episodes worsen HAAF, at least transiently, thus perpetuating a vicious cycle.
- Severe hypoglycemia requires prompt treatment with oral or parenteral glucose or glucagon, but the best treatment is prevention of future episodes.

INTRODUCTION

Because of their devastating long-term effects, the chronic complications of diabetes receive the bulk of attention in both clinical practice and the literature. However, the acute complications of diabetes also have devastating consequences and because of their emergent nature require prompt recognition and competent management. These complications are diabetic ketoacidosis (DKA), hyperosmolar hyperglycemic state (HHS), also known as hyperosmolar hyperglycemic nonketotic state, and hypoglycemia. They represent extremes in the spectrum of dysglycemia. This review provides current clinically relevant information on the epidemiology, pathogenesis, causes, clinical presentation, and management of these conditions.

Physician Assistant Program, Nova Southeastern University, 3200 South University Drive, Terry Building 1258, Ft Lauderdale, FL 33328-2018, USA
E-mail address: hfeldman@nova.edu

Physician Assist Clin 5 (2020) 191–211
https://doi.org/10.1016/j.cpha.2019.12.001
2405-7991/20/© 2019 Elsevier Inc. All rights reserved.

DIABETIC KETOACIDOSIS
Definition

National registries and observational studies have used somewhat different definitions of DKA.[1,2] However, a composite definition based on the salient biochemical features of DKA is that it is a state of absolute or relative insulin deficiency characterized by the following:

- Hyperglycemia (blood glucose usually >250 mg/dL)
- Metabolic acidosis (arterial pH <7.3 and/or bicarbonate <15mEq/L)
- Ketosis (ketonemia and ketonuria)

Epidemiology

DKA is most commonly associated with type 1 diabetes mellitus (T1DM). However, about one-third of DKA cases occur in type 2 diabetes (T2DM) under stressful conditions and as a presenting manifestation of a disorder called ketosis-prone diabetes mellitus (KPDM).[3] DKA is the presenting manifestation of diabetes in about 30% of children, less in adults, and most often because of some precipitating cause in patients with established disease.[4–6]

DKA is more common in young patients, especially children and adolescents. National registries and observational studies indicate that DKA is the presenting manifestation in 20% to 30% of youth with T1DM, with younger age and ethnic minority associated with higher prevalence rates[7] (**Fig. 1**). The Environmental Determinants of Diabetes in the Young study showed that genetic screening in early infancy coupled with intensive parental education and serial testing for islet cell autoantibodies in children at risk for T1DM can reduce the prevalence of DKA compared with conventional care.[1]

Age-adjusted hospitalization and mortality rates for DKA have shown divergent trends in the United States since the year 2000. Hospitalizations were relatively flat

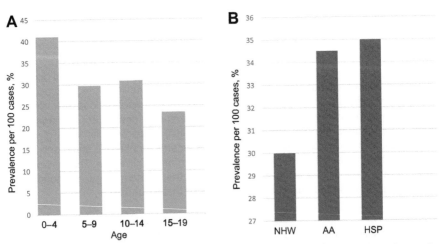

Fig. 1. (A) Prevalence of DKA in type 1 diabetes by age. (B) Prevalence of DKA in type 1 diabetes by ethnicity. Data are from 2008 to 2010. AA, African-American; HSP, hispanic; NHW, non-hispanic white. (*Adapted from* Dabelea D, Rewers A, Stafford JM, et al. Trends in the prevalence of ketoacidosis at diabetes diagnosis: The SEARCH for diabetes in Youth Study. Pediatrics 2014;133:e938-945.)

from 2000 to 2009 but increased thereafter to 2014. In contrast, mortalities declined steadily during the entire period to less than 1%[8] (**Fig. 2**). The reasons for the increase in hospitalizations for DKA are not known. Possible contributing factors include lack of standardized case definitions of DKA, the inclusion of "euglycemic DKA" seen with the new sodium-glucose cotransporter 2 (SGLT2) inhibitors for treating T2DM, and lower thresholds of disease severity prompting hospitalization. The lower threshold for hospitalization may also account for the decrease in DKA in-hospital mortality, although other proposed factors for the decline are better understanding of DKA pathophysiology and application of DKA treatment guidelines.[2,8] Nonetheless, although the overall mortality is less than 1%, the mortality is substantially worse at the extremes of age.[3,4]

Pathophysiology

Biochemical mechanisms

Under normal circumstances, blood glucose concentration is regulated by the opposing functions of insulin and glucagon. In the postprandial state, as blood glucose levels increase, insulin is secreted from beta cells in the pancreas. Insulin maintains normoglycemia by decreasing hepatic glucose production through inhibition of glycogenolysis and gluconeogenesis and by increasing glucose uptake in skeletal muscle and adipose tissue. In the latter, insulin inhibits lipolysis. Insulin also inhibits glucagon secretion from alpha cells in the pancreas.[9]

DKA develops when there is insulin deficiency combined with insulin resistance created by increased levels of counterregulatory hormones that oppose insulin. These hormones include glucagon, catecholamines, cortisol, and growth hormone. All contribute, but glucagon is most responsible for the hyperglycemia and ketoacidosis. Insulin deficiency and glucagon excess result in release of fatty acids from adipose

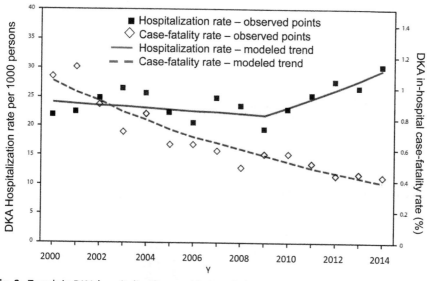

Fig. 2. Trends in DKA hospitalizations and in-hospital mortality–United States, 2000 to 2014. Symbols indicate observed points; lines indicate modeled trends. All trend lines were significant at a P value of less than 0.05. (*Reproduced from* Benoit SR, Zhang Y, Geiss LS, et al. Trends in diabetic ketoacidosis hospitalizations and in-hospital mortality — United States, 2000–2014. MMWR Morb Mortal Wkly Rep 2018; 67:362-365.)

tissue that go to the liver, where they are oxidized to ketoacids (beta-hydroxybutyric acid and acetoacetic acid, referred to as ketone bodies). The decreased metabolism and clearance of these ketone bodies also contribute to ketoacidosis. Glycosuria and ketonuria, which obligate water and electrolyte loss, lead to hypovolemia and decreased kidney function that further worsen the hyperglycemia and metabolic acidosis. Hyperosmolality results from dehydration, hyperglycemia, and ketonemia.

Fig. 3 is a schematic algorithm showing major contributors to the pathogenesis of DKA. More detailed discussions of the biochemical pathways and mechanisms involved in the pathogenesis of DKA can be found in Nyenwe and Kitabchi,[3] Powers and colleagues,[10] and Qiu and colleagues.[11]

Ketosis-prone type 2 diabetes mellitus

Although DKA is seen mostly in patients with T1DM, about one-third of DKA episodes occur in patients with T2DM who have a heterogeneous syndrome known as KPDM.[12,13] This entity was first reported from Africa in the 1960s, but more than half of African Americans with a new diagnosis of DKA have clinical and metabolic features of T2DM during follow-up.[13] KPDM is also more common among Hispanics and other minority ethnic groups than among Caucasians. **Table 1** compares type 1 with type 2 KPDM patients with DKA.

"Euglycemic" DKA owing to sodium-glucose cotransporter-2 inhibitors

Although hyperglycemia in DKA is defined by a glucose level greater than 250 mg/dL, rare cases of "euglycemic" DKA with normal to only modestly elevated glucose levels have sporadically appeared in the literature since 1973.[16] These early cases were seen in patients with T1DM most commonly in conjunction with food (especially carbohydrate) restriction, impaired gluconeogenesis owing to alcohol abuse, partial treatment of DKA, and pregnancy.[16–19] However, because the first-in-class SGLT2 inhibitor, canagliflozin, was introduced in 2013, this variant of DKA has been reported more frequently. SGLT2 inhibitors inhibit sodium and glucose reabsorption in the proximal

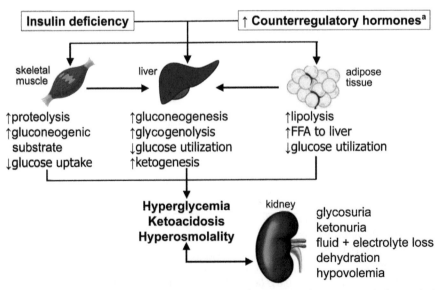

Fig. 3. Pathogenesis of DKA. [a] Counterregulatory hormones: glucagon, cortisol, catecholamines, growth hormone. FFA, free fatty acids. (*Adapted from* Kitabchi 2009.)

Table 1
Differences between diabetic ketoacidosis in type 1 and type 2 ketosis-prone diabetes mellitus

	Type 1 Diabetes	KPDM
Age at presentation	Childhood, adolescence	Adolescence, adulthood
Body habitus	Lean	Predominantly overweight to obese
Ethnicity	Predominantly Caucasian	Predominantly black, Latino, and other minorities
Family history of type 2 diabetes	No	Frequent
HLA-associated genetic markers	Common	Uncommon
Islet cell autoantibodies	Present in 100%	Uncommon
Beta-cell reserve	Absent in 100%	Common
Recurrent DKA episodes	Common	Rare if antibody (−) and beta-cell reserve (+)
Insulin-independent at 6–12 mo after DKA	No	Common if antibody (−) and beta-cell reserve (+)

Data from Refs.[3,13–15]

tubule of the kidney, thereby producing glycosuria and an osmotic diuresis. Within 2 years after their introduction, reports of euglycemic DKA appeared in the literature, prompting the Food and Drug Administration (FDA) to issue a warning.[18,20] Euglycemic DKA owing to SGLT2 inhibitors has been reported in patients with T2DM, and especially in T1DM, when these medications were used off-label. Median time to onset is 43 days with a range from 1 day to 1 year. Because of the absence of marked hyperglycemia, the diagnosis is often missed by both patients and clinicians despite classic symptoms of DKA.[18] Patients taking these medications, especially those with T1DM, should monitor their blood ketones whenever they feel ill.[18] If positive, they should notify their health care provider even if their blood glucose level is not severely elevated. In addition, these drugs should be held during periods of fasting or very low carbohydrate intake, and ketogenic diets should be avoided.[11]

The most recent report of SGLT2 inhibitor-induced DKA comes from nationwide registries in Sweden and Denmark.[21] Using propensity score matching, the investigators compared the risk of adverse events in 17,213 new users of SGLT2 inhibitors with 17,213 new users of glucagon-like peptide-1 (GLP-1) receptor agonists. They found a 2-fold increased risk of DKA with SGLT2 inhibitors, although the absolute risk was small (1.1 vs 0.6 events per 1000 person-years). These results are similar to data from the United States as well as a large meta-analysis of randomized controlled trials and observational studies.[22,23]

The mechanisms of euglycemic DKA with SGLT2 inhibitors are not fully known, but those that have been suggested lead to 1 common endpoint: a high glucagon:insulin ratio that shifts substrate usage from carbohydrates to lipids, that favors lipolysis and ketogenesis, and away from hyperglycemia.[11,18]

Not yet FDA approved is sotagliflozin, the first SGLT1 and 2 inhibitor that blocks glucose reabsorption in both the kidney and the intestine. In a meta-analysis of 6 randomized trials, this drug lowered glycemic variability and risk of hypoglycemia in patients with T1DM, but significantly raised the risk for DKA (18 vs 5 per 1000 patients), especially in patients with A1c less than 8%.[24] Whether this or other drugs in this new class will gain approval is uncertain because of concern about DKA.

Precipitating Factors

The most common precipitating causes of DKA are omission or inadequate dosing of insulin, acute illness, and new-onset diabetes.[4,25] Of these, poor adherence to insulin therapy has emerged as the leading cause, especially in patients with recurrent DKA.[4,6] Omission of insulin doses is particularly common among adolescents. Reasons for nonadherence, especially among the young, include psychological stress and depression, eating disorders, fear of weight gain, fear of hypoglycemia, and/or rebellion against authority.[26] Additional reasons include affordability of insulin, misuse of insulin pumps, and unintentional underdosing, especially during acute illness.[3,6,27] Acute illness is the second most common cause of DKA, especially pulmonary and urinary tract infections and illnesses that are associated with vomiting and dehydration[3,4,6] (**Box 1**).

Clinical Presentation

Symptoms and signs

The symptoms and signs of DKA develop rapidly, usually over 24 hours or less. They are the result of hyperglycemia, acidosis, and fluid and electrolyte losses. Hyperglycemia causes polyuria from glucose-induced osmotic diuresis and polydipsia in response to the urinary water loss. Metabolic acidosis causes hyperventilation with deep (Kussmaul) respirations, which is the compensatory respiratory response to the low blood pH. Acidosis also causes anorexia, nausea and vomiting, and neurologic features ranging from lethargy to obtundation and coma depending on severity. Although hyperosmolality can also cause neurologic symptoms, it does so at levels greater than 320 mOsm/kg, which are seen in HHS but in only about 30% of patients

---

Box 1
Precipitating causes of diabetic ketoacidosis

Inadequate insulin dosing or noncompliance

New-onset diabetes mellitus

Acute illness
- Infections (especially pulmonary and urinary tract)
- Acute pancreatitis
- Acute myocardial infarction
- Cerebrovascular accident
- Trauma (physical or psychological)

Drugs
- Corticosteroids
- Thiazides
- SGLT2 inhibitors
- Sympathomimetics (eg, terbutaline)
- Atypical antipsychotics (eg, clozapine, olanzapine)
- Amphetamines
- Cocaine
- Alcohol abuse
- Cannabis

Endocrine disorders
- Acromegaly
- Pheochromocytoma

Data from Refs.[3,28]

with DKA. Accumulation of acetone causes a fruity odor to the breath. Fluid and electrolyte losses cause weight loss and signs of intravascular volume contraction and dehydration, including tachycardia, hypotension, and decreased skin turgor.[3,4,25]

Another clinical feature of DKA is abdominal pain that can be mistaken for other pathologic conditions, such as acute pancreatitis or even a surgical emergency. In 1 series, abdominal pain occurred in 86 of 189 patients (46%) and strongly correlated with the severity of acidosis.[29] This finding suggests that abdominal pain in the absence of severe acidosis should prompt investigation for a cause other than DKA.

A major clinical complication of DKA that occurs primarily in children is cerebral edema. The prevalence is only 0.3% to 0.9% of cases, but it is the leading cause of mortality from DKA in this population.[30,31] Symptoms typically develop within 12 hours after starting therapy, but can appear before treatment.[32] For a detailed discussion of cerebral injury in children with DKA, see the review by Glaser.[33]

The severity of DKA is determined by the degree of acidemia and extent of neurologic impairment and not by the severity of hyperglycemia, which may be mild (**Table 2**).

Laboratory evaluation

The initial laboratory evaluation should include a chemistry panel, urinalysis, serum and urine ketones, arterial blood gas, complete blood count, and other clinically indicated tests to identify precipitating factors. With the exception of euglycemic DKA, blood glucose levels are greater than 250 mg/dL but less than 800 mg/dL, averaging 300 to 500 mg/dL. Until stable, glucose should be checked hourly, and electrolytes, renal function, and venous pH should be checked every 2 to 4 hours. The hallmark laboratory abnormality in DKA is ketoacidosis owing to the accumulation of acetoacetate and beta-hydroxybutyrate, which are acid anions, and acetone, which is a ketone but not an acid and therefore does not contribute to the acidosis. The major ketone produced in DKA is beta-hydroxybutyrate. However, the urine dipsticks for ketones measure only acetoacetate and acetone, which underestimate the degree of ketosis. Moreover, as ketosis is corrected with treatment, beta-hydroxybutyrate is converted to acetoacetate and acetone. The urine dipstick will then give the false impression that the ketosis is worsening. Therefore, the best test to assess the degree of ketosis and the response to treatment is serum beta-hydroxybutyrate, which is available as a point-of-care test.[34]

The best method to assess the severity of metabolic acidosis is the blood pH (arterial or venous). However, the anion gap, calculated from the venous chemistry panel, can also provide useful information on the degree of ketoacid accumulation. The anion gap (reference range 3–10 mEq/L) is equal to: serum sodium – (serum chloride + bicarbonate). In DKA, the gap is often greater than 20 mEq/L.

Table 2			
Severity-based diagnostic criteria for diabetic ketoacidosis			
	Mild	**Moderate**	**Severe**
Arterial pH	7.25–7.30	7.00–7.24	<7.00
Serum bicarbonate (mEq/L)	15–18	10–14.9	<10
Mental status	Alert	Alert to drowsy	Stupor or coma

Data from Umpierrez G, Korytkiwski M. Diabetic emergencies – ketoacidosis, hyperglycaemic hyperosmolar state and hypoglycaemia. Nat Rev Endocrinol 2016;12:222-32.

The chemistry panel also provides other critical data. It can be used to calculate the effective plasma osmolality, which equals [2 × sodium (mEq/L) + [glucose (mg/dL) ÷ 18].[34] The shift of water from the intracellular to extracellular compartment owing to the hyperglycemia will lower the serum sodium concentration. Therefore, a normal or high sodium concentration implies a significant degree of dehydration. A "corrected" sodium concentration that accounts for the water shift can be obtained by adding 2 mEq/L to the measured sodium concentration for each 100 mg/dL increase in glucose concentration above normal. An intracellular to extracellular shift also occurs with potassium and phosphorus. Despite uniform deficits owing to urinary losses, serum potassium and phosphorus levels may be normal or even increased. The intracellular shift that occurs with treatment reveals the true deficits. Blood urea nitrogen (BUN) elevation, disproportionate to creatinine, correlates with the degree of hypovolemia, whereas comparable elevation of creatinine indicates acute kidney injury.[34]

Leukocytosis is common in DKA and is due to the increase in catecholamines. It usually is ≤15,000/mL and correlates with the degree of ketonemia. Higher levels and/or more than 10% bands should prompt a search for an underlying infection.[26]

Nonspecific elevations of serum amylase, usually of salivary origin, and serum lipase are often seen in DKA, making it difficult to determine if acute pancreatitis is also present. A contrast-enhanced computed tomographic scan can rule out this possibility.[35]

Treatment

The treatment objectives in DKA are as follows:

- Correct hypovolemia with intravenous (IV) fluids (**Box 2**)
- Correct electrolyte disturbances, especially potassium (**Box 3**)
- Correct hyperglycemia (**Box 4**)
- Correct ketoacidosis
- Identify and treat precipitating cause or causes and comorbid conditions

Correction of hypovolemia

The first step in treating DKA is to correct the extracellular volume and free water deficits. Replacement should begin with rapid IV infusion of isotonic saline to restore intravascular volume. Subsequent fluid replacement will depend on the corrected serum sodium concentration and state of rehydration as assessed by hemodynamic monitoring and urine output[3] (see **Box 2**).

Correction of electrolyte disturbances

All patients with DKA have potassium deficits that can reach several hundred milliequivalents. However, the serum potassium is often normal or elevated because of insulin deficiency, acidemia, and hypertonicity. If hypokalemia is present, this must be corrected before giving insulin because insulin drives potassium into cells and could cause life-threatening cardiac arrhythmias[3,26] (see **Box 3**).

Phosphate deficits also are common. However, replacement is not recommended unless severe hypophosphatemia (<1 mg/dL) develops. Phosphate replacement can cause hypocalcemia and hypomagnesemia, and clinical trials have not shown any benefit in clinical outcomes with routine phosphate replacement.[37]

Correction of hyperglycemia

Insulin should be started promptly or after hypokalemia, if present, is corrected. Glucose should be checked hourly, and electrolytes, BUN, creatinine, and pH should be checked every 2 to 4 hours until stable.[26] Because of variability in the severity of

---

Box 2
Volume and free water replacement in adults with diabetic ketoacidosis

For severe hypovolemia with cardiovascular compromise (shock)
• Rapid IV infusion of several liters of isotonic (0.9%) saline[a]

For hypovolemia without shock
• IV isotonic (0.9%) saline at 15 to 20 mL/kg per hour (~1–1.5 L/h) for first few hours[a]
  ○ Most patients will need at least 3 L in first 5 hours

After intravascular volume is restored
• Calculate corrected serum sodium concentration (see text)
• If corrected sodium concentration is normal or high, give one-half isotonic (0.45%) saline at 250 to 500 mL per hour, depending on degree of water deficit[a]
• If corrected sodium concentration is low, continue isotonic saline until normal
  ○ Sodium concentration will increase as hyperglycemia is corrected
• Water deficits should be corrected in the first 24 hours[b]

When plasma glucose decreases to ~200 mg/dL
• Switch IV fluid to 5% dextrose in 0.45% saline

[a] In patients with heart failure, the rate and amount of fluid will have to be reduced. [b] Water deficit = (0.6)(body weight in kg) × (1 − [corrected sodium/140]).

Data from Refs.[3,26,36]

---

hyperglycemia, treatment should be individualized. Mild to moderate DKA can be treated with subcutaneous rapid-acting insulin analogues, but severe DKA is treated with continuous IV infusion of regular insulin. An initial bolus dose is no longer considered necessary[3,26] (see **Box 4**).

In a recently reported before-and-after study, a less-intensive insulin regimen resulted in shorter hospital stays, less hypoglycemia, and less glycemic variability. The initial infusion rate was 0.05 to 0.1 units/kg/h; dose titration was limited to 25% increments to lower blood glucose by only 26 to 50 mg/dL/h, and target blood glucose was increased to 200 to 300 mg/dL. This regimen requires further validation because the study was retrospective, small (201 patients), and conducted in a single medical center.[38]

Correction of metabolic acidosis
Correction of metabolic acidosis with sodium bicarbonate therapy is unnecessary in most patients. Insulin and volume expansion will suffice to shut off production of

---

Box 3
Potassium replacement in adults with diabetic ketoacidosis

For serum potassium (K+) less than 3.3 mEq/L
• Hold insulin
• Give potassium chloride 20 to 40 mEq/h IV until K+ is greater than 3.3 mEq/L

For serum K+ 3.3 to 5.3 mEq/L
• Give potassium chloride 20 to 30 mEq/L of IV fluid to maintain serum K+ between 4 and 5 mEq/L

For serum K+ greater than 5.3 mEq/L
• Do not give K+
• Check serum K+ every 2 hours
• Initiate K+ replacement when serum K+ decreases to 5 to 5.2 mEq/L

Data from Refs.[3,36]

Box 4
Insulin therapy in adults with diabetic ketoacidosis

Uncomplicated mild to moderate DKA
- Rapid-acting insulin (lispro, aspart) 0.3 unit/kg subcutaneous (sq) followed by hourly 0.1 unit/kg sq until glucose less than 250 mg/dL, then 0.05 units/kg sq hourly until DKA resolves[a]

Severe DKA
- Start continuous IV infusion of regular insulin at 0.1 to 0.2 units/kg/h
- Increase hourly rate by 20% to 50% to lower blood glucose by 50 to 70 mg/dL/h
- Decrease rate to 0.02 to 0.05 units/kg/h when glucose reaches 200 mg/dL
- Continue infusion until ketoacidosis resolves and glucose is less than 200 mg/dL
- Start multidose sq maintenance insulin and discontinue IV infusion 2 hours later if patient is able to eat; otherwise, continue IV insulin and fluids.

[a] DKA resolution = Blood glucose less than 200 mg/dL + 2 of the following: serum bicarbonate $\geq$15 mEq/L, venous pH >7.3, anion gap $\leq$12 mEq/L. However, bicarbonate concentration may not be reliable after the first 6 hours because of hyperchloremia from IV saline infusion.

Data from Refs.[3,26]

---

ketoacids and promote their urinary excretion. Although controversial, bicarbonate therapy may be beneficial in the following 2 groups of patients with DKA:

- Patients with pH $\leq$6.9: Severe acidemia decreases cardiac contractility and cardiac output and causes vasodilatation, all of which can aggravate the hypotensive effect of hypovolemia. It also predisposes to cardiac arrhythmias.[39]
- Patients with severe hyperkalemia (>6.4 mEq/L): Bicarbonate drives potassium into cells.

HYPEROSMOLAR HYPERGLYCEMIC STATE
Definition

HHS is characterized by more severe hyperglycemia, hyperosmolality, and dehydration than is seen in DKA and by the absence of ketoacidosis.[26]

Epidemiology

HHS most often occurs in geriatric, often institutionalized, patients with T2DM (average age 60; range 57–69).[40] However, HHS does occur in younger adults and even in pediatric patients with either T1DM or T2DM.[41] In these patients it often presents as mixed DKA-HHS rather than as HHS alone.[42] HHS occurs more commonly in ethnic minorities, probably because of the greater prevalence of T2DM. Although HHS accounts for less than 1% of diabetes-related hospital admissions, its mortality of 5% to 20% is 10 times higher than the mortality of DKA. This mortality is due to the older age, greater comorbidities, and more severe hyperglycemia, hyperosmolality, and dehydration seen in HHS patients.[26,43]

Pathogenesis

Like DKA, HHS is due to insulin deficiency accompanied by increased glucagon and other counterregulatory hormones. However, the deficiency of insulin is less severe in HHS than in DKA. Also, glucagon excess is less in HHS than in DKA. Because less insulin is required to suppress lipolysis and ketogenesis than gluconeogenesis, the higher insulin/glucagon ratio limits ketogenesis and accounts for the absence of ketoacidosis.[26] Hyperosmolality may also inhibit lipolysis and protect against ketoacidosis.[44]

Precipitating Factors

HHS is precipitated by many of the same factors as DKA, especially acute stress and concomitant illness, with infection as the leading cause (see **Box 1**). However, there are some differences in precipitating factors compared with DKA,[4,40,43] as follows:

- HHS patients usually have established T2DM; undiagnosed or new-onset diabetes is less common.
- Omission of oral hypoglycemic agents is more common than omission of insulin.
- Advanced age-related illnesses are more common (eg, stroke, myocardial infarction).
- Reduced fluid intake plays a greater role because of an age-related decrease in thirst perception and limited access to water because of conditions such as dementia or stroke, or being bedridden.

Clinical Presentation

Symptoms and signs

Symptoms develop over several days to weeks. The longer duration contributes to the more severe hyperglycemia, hyperosmolality, and dehydration compared with DKA. Although polyuria, polydipsia, weakness, and weight loss occur, neurologic manifestations, ranging from lethargy to coma and seizures, dominate the clinical presentation because of the marked hyperosmolality (>320 mOsm/kg). There is a linear relationship between osmolality and degree of obtundation. Water deficits of 6 to 10 L cause signs of dehydration (hypotension, dry oral mucosa, decreased skin turgor). In contrast to DKA, nausea, vomiting, and abdominal pain are uncommon, and Kussmaul respirations are absent.[26]

Laboratory evaluation

Table 3 compares the key differentiating laboratory findings in HHS versus DKA. However, it also reflects the important fact that there is overlap in laboratory findings in about a third of patients.[4,10,26]

Although electrolyte values are variable, serum sodium concentrations tend to be higher in HHS because of the greater water losses; the elevated serum sodium indicates severe dehydration. Likewise, the greater volume losses tend to increase the BUN, creatinine, and BUN/creatinine ratio higher than in DKA.[26,43]

Treatment

With the exception of correcting acidosis, the principles of treating HHS are much the same as for DKA (see **Boxes 2–4**). However, there are some differences in detail, as follows:

- Fluid resuscitation in HHS may have to be more vigorous because of the greater degree of volume loss and likelihood of hypotension at presentation. The average loss is 9 L, as compared with less than 6 L in DKA.[43]
- It is important to restore intravascular volume before insulin administration because insulin will shift both glucose and water into cells, thereby worsening hypovolemia and hypotension.[43]
- Close attention should be paid to the rate of decrease in plasma osmolality because too rapid of a reduction (>3 mOsm/kg/h) may cause cerebral edema. The water deficit should be corrected over 1 to 2 days with hypotonic fluid.[10,36,43]
- As with DKA, slow continuous IV infusion of insulin at 0.1 units/kg/h is given. However, the rate is reduced when plasma glucose levels decrease to 300 mg/dL instead of 200 mg/dL, and the initial plasma glucose target is between

Table 3
Laboratory findings in hyperosmolar hyperglycemic state versus diabetic ketoacidosis

	HHS	DKA
Plasma glucose (mg/dL)	>600–1200	>250 (usually <600)
Serum osmolality (mOsm/kg)	>320–380	Variable (usually <320)
Arterial pH	>7.30[a]	≤7.30
Serum bicarbonate (mEq/L)	Normal to slightly decreased[a]	<15–18
Anion gap	Normal to slightly increased[a]	Increased
Serum ketones	Negative to small[b]	Positive
Urine ketones	Negative to small[b]	Positive
Serum amylase	Normal	Often elevated

[a] Mild anion-gap metabolic acidosis may occur due to increased lactic acid or renal failure.
[b] Mild ketosis may occur due to starvation.
Data from Refs.[4,10,26]

250 and 300 mg/dL instead of 150 to 200 mg/dL until the patient is mentally alert. This more conservative correction of hyperglycemia is done to prevent a too rapid decline in plasma osmolality.[43]

Differential Diagnosis

Because of overlap, a mixed DKA-HHS presentation may occur.[26,42,43] In addition, these 2 disorders must be differentiated from other causes of hyperglycemia, ketosis, metabolic acidosis, and metabolic encephalopathy that also may overlap or coexist with either DKA or HHS. **Fig. 4** depicts these interactions.

HYPOGLYCEMIA

This section is limited to a discussion of iatrogenic hypoglycemia related to diabetes treatment. Other causes of hypoglycemia are beyond the scope of this review.

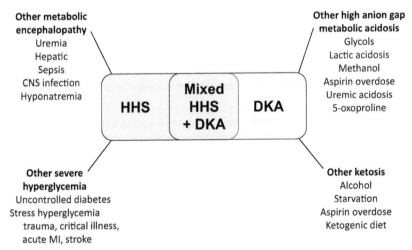

Fig. 4. Differential diagnosis of DKA and HHS. MI, myocardial infarction. (*Adapted from* Kitabchi AE and Nyenwe EA. Hyperglycemic crises in diabetes mellitus: Diabetic ketoacidosis and hyperglycemic hyperosmolar state. Endocrinol Metab Clin N Am2006;35:725-751.)

Definition

Because the blood glucose threshold at which hypoglycemic symptoms appear varies between patients and within individual patients over time, as well as with antecedent glycemic control, there is no single level that defines hypoglycemia. Rather, current consensus defines 3 glucose thresholds that correlate with increasing degrees of harm from hypoglycemia[45] (**Table 4**).

Epidemiology

Hypoglycemia is the most common serious iatrogenic complication of diabetes.[48] However, the true frequency of this complication is difficult to determine from the literature because of differences in definition, study design, and patient characteristics. Moreover, most asymptomatic (biochemical) or mildly symptomatic episodes are not reported or incorrectly interpreted by patients.[48,49]

The best data come from large prospective population-based studies because randomized controlled trial data are less generalizable. One such study is a recent 4-week prospective study of 27,585 adults with type 1 and type 2 diabetes conducted in 24 countries[50] (**Table 5**). Although other studies have yielded different rates, they all indicate that hypoglycemia occurs very frequently.[4,48,49,51–53]

Although the rate per person is less in T2DM, there are far more patients with T2DM than T1DM. Thus, most hypoglycemia encountered in clinical practice occurs in patients with T2DM.

As much as 6% to 10% of deaths in T1DM are associated with hypoglycemia.[54] Severe hypoglycemia is associated with a 3.4-fold higher 5-year mortality compared with mild or no hypoglycemia.[55] Cardiovascular morbidities, especially arrhythmias, may explain much of this association.[4,56]

Pathogenesis

Hypoglycemia in diabetes is due to a combination of therapeutic hyperinsulinemia and impaired counterregulatory mechanisms that protect against a decrease in blood glucose.[57] Excess insulin replacement is the culprit in T1DM and in insulin-requiring T2DM. Insulin secretagogues, especially sulfonylureas and to a lesser extent meglitinides, also cause hypoglycemia in T2DM. Of the sulfonylureas, glyburide, because of its longer half-life, causes hypoglycemia much more often than glipizide.[58] Other

Table 4		
Definition of hypoglycemia based on level of harm		
	Glucose (mg/dL)[a]	**Comments on Glucose Level[a]**
Level 1 (Alert)	≤70 to >54	Lower limit of nondiabetic fasting range and threshold for normal neuroendocrine response May be asymptomatic or mildly symptomatic Alerts patient to take action
Level 2 (Action)	≤54	Neuroglycopenic symptoms likely. Immediate action needed
Level 3 (Assistance)	No specific glucose threshold	Severe symptoms. Altered mental and/or physical status requiring assistance from others

[a] Values and comments are based on laboratory blood glucose measurements (gold standard). Capillary (glucose meters) and interstitial fluid (continuous glucose monitor) readings may differ from laboratory values but can still be used to guide action.
Data from Refs.[45–47]

Table 5			
Frequency of hypoglycemia in diabetes			
	Hypoglycemic Events per Patient per Year		
	Overall	Nocturnal	Severe
Type 1 diabetes	73.3	11.3	4.9
Type 2 diabetes	19.3	3.7	2.5

Data from Khunti K, Alsifri s, Aronson M, et al. Rates and predictors of hypoglycemia in 27,585 people from 24 countries with insulin-treated type 1 and type 2 diabetes: the global HAT study. Diabetes Obes Metab 2016;18:907-15.

drugs used in T2DM, including metformin, GLP-1 receptor agonists, SGLT2, and dipeptidyl peptidase-4 inhibitors, do not cause hypoglycemia unless combined with insulin or insulin secretagogues.[59]

In addition to iatrogenic hypoglycemia, impaired counterregulatory mechanisms contribute to the development and recurrence of hypoglycemia. First, loss of beta-cell insulin secretion blunts alpha-cell glucagon secretion in response to hypoglycemia. Second, the resulting hypoglycemia impairs both components of the sympathoadrenal response to hypoglycemia, known as hypoglycemia-associated autonomic failure (HAAF): (1) epinephrine and (2) sympathetic neural response. Loss of the epinephrine response prevents restoration of normoglycemia, and loss of the neural response prevents recognition of hypoglycemia (hypoglycemia unawareness). Recent exercise and sleep also contribute to HAAF; the former suppresses the epinephrine response and the latter contributes to nocturnal hypoglycemia, which is more commonly associated with cardiac arrhythmias than is daytime hypoglycemia.[4] Moreover, the worse the hypoglycemia, the more deficient is the sympathoadrenal response. This vicious cycle favors recurrent severe hypoglycemia (**Fig. 5**).[60]

It is worth noting HAAF is not permanent. Avoidance of hypoglycemia for as little as 2 to 3 weeks restores responsiveness to epinephrine and reverses hypoglycemic unawareness.[57] Conversely, the risk of severe hypoglycemia is substantially increased

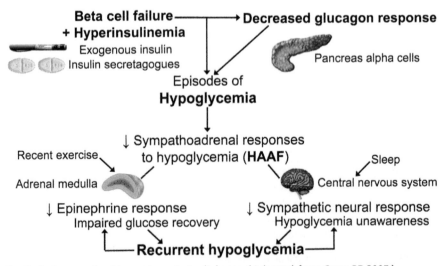

Fig. 5. Pathogenesis of hypoglycemia in diabetes. (*Adapted from* Cryer PE 2005.)

by antecedent asymptomatic hypoglycemia as well as by tight glycemic control (A1c ≤6.5%).[61–63] Paradoxically, poor glycemic control (A1c ≥9%) also predisposes to severe hypoglycemia, perhaps because of intensive efforts to lower blood glucose.[64]

Risk Factors for Iatrogenic Hypoglycemia

Risk factors for hypoglycemia related to treatment of diabetes fall into the 2 following categories[4,27,46,47]:

1. Mismatch between insulin or insulin secretagogue dosing versus glucose availability
   - Excessive or ill-timed dosing
     o Intensive glycemic therapy (targeting low A1c levels)
     o Poor coordination of dosing with food delivery
     o Wrong type of insulin (incorrect amount of basal and/or bolus insulin)
     o Abrupt reduction in nutritional intake
     o Gastroparesis or intestinal malabsorption of glucose
     o Weight loss (eg, dieting or postbariatric surgery → increased insulin sensitivity)
     o Vigorous exercise (increased glucose utilization)
   - Decreased glucose production
     o Heavy alcohol ingestion
     o Liver failure
   - Decreased insulin clearance
     o Kidney failure
2. HAAF
   - Long duration of diabetes (severe beta-cell failure impairs glucagon response)
   - Recurring hypoglycemia, especially recent antecedent hypoglycemia
   - Hypoglycemia unawareness (prevents detection and behavioral response)
   - Prior exercise or sleep (blunt sympathoadrenal responses)
   - Advanced age

Clinical Presentation

Symptoms and signs

The acute symptoms and signs of hypoglycemia are due to the neurogenic (autonomic) responses to hypoglycemia and the consequences of decreased delivery of glucose to the brain (neuroglycopenia).[47]

1. Neurogenic
   - Catecholamine (norepinephrine)-mediated: Palpitations, tremors, anxiety, tachycardia, cardiac arrhythmias
   - Cholinergic (acetylcholine)-mediated: Sweating, hunger, paresthesias, nausea
2. Neuroglycopenic
   - Dizziness, weakness, impaired concentration, and confusion that progresses with more profound hypoglycemia to drowsiness, delirium, seizures, and coma

Long-term consequences result from repeated episodes of hypoglycemia. These consequences include impaired cognitive function, falls, absenteeism from work, impaired quality of life, fear, anxiety and depression, emergency department visits, and hospitalizations.[4,53,54,65–67]

Treatment

Treatment depends on the state of consciousness of the patient and ability to take oral carbohydrates (**Table 6**). Patients and family members should be educated on recognizing and responding to symptoms of hypoglycemia, including how to administer glucagon. Insulin-dependent patients should carry a glucagon kit and either glucose tablets or carbohydrate source.

Until recently, glucagon was marketed solely as a lyophilized powder that had to be reconstituted with a diluent before it could be injected. In July 2019, the FDA approved a device that delivers 3 mg of glucagon intranasally. It has shown noninferiority to intramuscular glucagon.[68] Another device, approved in September 2019, is a glucagon pen that delivers glucagon subcutaneously without the need for reconstitution.[69]

Prevention

The occurrence and fear of hypoglycemia are major limiting factors in preventing long-term optimal glycemic control.[56,70] Therefore, preventing hypoglycemia is crucial to the successful management of diabetes. The report of a workgroup of the American Diabetes Association and the Endocrine Society describes approaches that can prevent hypoglycemia.[46] It also provides 2 helpful aids for patients and clinicians: A questionnaire that guides patients and their families on monitoring, recognizing, preventing, and treating hypoglycemia, and a provider checklist designed to verify that the clinician has asked the correct questions and made the best recommendations for

Table 6
Treatment of hypoglycemia

Clinical State	Acute Treatment Options	Follow-Through Treatment
Alert and mildly symptomatic	1. 15–20 g of rapidly absorbed glucose. Examples: • 1 tbs sugar, jelly, honey, or corn syrup • ½ cup of sweetened fruit juice or regular soda • 6–8 hard candies • 4–5 saltine crackers • 2 tbs of raisins 2. 3–4 glucose tablets (4 g each)[a] 3. Glucagon 0.5–1 mg sq or intramuscularly (IM)[b]	Recheck blood glucose in 15 min and repeat dose if ≤70 mg/dL Eat a snack or meal within an hour to prevent recurrence Avoid critical tasks until stable (eg, driving)
Stuporous or comatose (requires third-party assistance)	1. Out of hospital • Glucagon 0.5–1 mg sq or IM, or 3 mg intranasally 2. In hospital • 10–25 g of IV dextrose • Glucagon sq or IM if IV access is not available[b]	Continuous blood glucose monitoring and IV dextrose or food (if able to eat) until effect of insulin or insulin secretagogue wears off

[a] Use only glucose tablets for patients on alpha-glucosidase inhibitors because these drugs slow down digestion of dietary disaccharides.
[b] Avoid glucagon in glycogen-depleted patients (eg, with prolonged fasting or adrenal insufficiency, or after heavy alcohol use or vigorous sustained exercise).
Data from American Diabetes Association. 6. Glycemic Targets: Standards of Medical Care in Diabetes—2019. Diabetes Care 2019 Jan; 42(Supplement 1): S61-S70. https://doi.org/10.2337/dc19-S006.

managing hypoglycemia. Although details of the report are beyond the scope of this review, a few key elements should be noted, as follows:

- Patient education is crucial. Patients should be taught how to adjust medications, diet, and exercise to maintain euglycemia.
- Frequent monitoring of blood glucose is essential for all patients with type 1 diabetes and hypoglycemia-prone type 2 diabetes. Continuous glucose monitors and sensor-augmented insulin pumps are making this task easier and have reduced the incidence of hypoglycemia.[71,72]
- Flexible insulin regimens that match bolus and basal insulin dosing to patients' eating and activity patterns are essential.
- Realistic, individualized glycemic (A1c) goals based on patients' comorbidities, propensity for hypoglycemia, and life expectancy are crucial.

Despite these measures, currently, hypoglycemia is a fact of life for all patients with T1DM and some patients with T2DM. However, it is hoped that technological advances, such as the artificial pancreas, may someday relieve patients of this debilitating complication.

DISCLOSURE

None.

REFERENCES

1. Larsson HE, Vehik K, Bell R, et al. Reduced prevalence of diabetic ketoacidosis at diagnosis of type 1 diabetes in young children participating in longitudinal follow-up. Diabetes Care 2011;34:2347–52.
2. Dhatariya KK. Why the definitions used to diagnose diabetic ketoacidosis should be standardized. Diabetes Res Clin Pract 2018;135:227–8.
3. Nyenwe EA, Kitabchi AE. The evolution of diabetic ketoacidosis: an update of its etiology, pathogenesis and management. Metabolism 2016;65:507–21.
4. Umpierrez G, Korytkiwski M. Diabetic emergencies–ketoacidosis, hyperglycaemic hyperosmolar state and hypoglycaemia. Nat Rev Endocrinol 2016;12: 222–32.
5. Klingensmith GJ, Tamborlane WV, Wood J, et al. Diabetic ketoacidosis at diabetes onset: still an all too common threat in youth. J Pediatr 2013;162:330–4.e1.
6. Randall L, Begovic J, Hudson M, et al. Recurrent diabetic ketoacidosis in inner-city minority patients. Diabetes Care 2011;34:1891–6.
7. Dabelea D, Rewers A, Stafford JM, et al. Trends in the prevalence of ketoacidosis at diabetes diagnosis: the SEARCH for diabetes in youth study. Pediatrics 2014; 133:e938–45.
8. Benoit SR, Zhang Y, Geiss LS, et al. Trends in diabetic ketoacidosis hospitalizations and in-hospital mortality–United States 2000-2014. MMWR Morb Mortal Wkly Rep 2018;67:362–5.
9. Powers AC, Niswender KD, Evans-Molina C. Diabetes mellitus: diagnosis, classification, and pathophysiology; regulation of glucose homeostasis. In: Jameson J, Fauci AS, Kasper DL, et al, editors. Harrison's principles of internal medicine. 20th edition. New York: McGraw-Hill; 2018. Subscription required to view. Available at: http://www.accessmedicine.com. Accessed February 12, 2019.
10. Powers AC, Niswender KD, Rickels MR. Diabetes mellitus: management and therapies; acute disorders related to severe hyperglycemia. In: Jameson J, Fauci AS, Kasper DL, et al, editors. Harrison's principles of internal medicine.

20th edition. New York: McGraw-Hill; 2018. Subscription required to view. Available at: http://www.accessmedicine.com. Accessed February 12, 2019.

11. Qiu H, Novikov A, Vallon V. Ketosis and diabetic ketoacidosis in response to SGLT2 inhibitors: basic mechanisms and therapeutic perspectives. Diabetes Metab Res Rev 2017;33(5):e2886.

12. Newton CA, Raskin P. Diabetic ketoacidosis in type 1 and type 2 diabetes mellitus. Arch Intern Med 2004;164:1925–31.

13. Vellanki P, Umpierrez GE. Diabetic ketoacidosis: a common debut of diabetes among African Americans with type 2 diabetes. Endocr Pract 2017;23:971–8.

14. Maldonado M, Hampe CS, Gaur LK, et al. Ketosis-prone diabetes: dissection of a heterogeneous syndrome using an immunogenic and β-cell functional classification, prospective analysis, and clinical outcomes. J Clin Endocrinol Metab 2003; 88:5090–8.

15. Umpierrez GE, Smiley D, Kitabchi AE. Narrative review: ketosis-prone type 2 diabetes mellitus. Ann Intern Med 2006;144:350–7.

16. Munro JF, Campbell LW, McCuish AC, et al. Euglycemic diabetic ketoacidosis. BMJ 1973;2:578–80.

17. Joseph F, Anderson L, Goenka N, et al. Starvation-induced true diabetic euglycemic ketoacidosis in severe depression. J Gen Intern Med 2008;24:129–31.

18. Peters AL, Buschur EO, Buse JB, et al. Euglycemic diabetic ketoacidosis: a potential complication of treatment with sodium-glucose cotransporter 2 inhibition. Diabetes Care 2015;38:1687–93.

19. Chico M, Levine SN, Lewis DF. Normoglycemic diabetic ketoacidosis in pregnancy. J Perinatol 2008;28:310–2.

20. FDA Drug Safety Communication. FDA warns that SGLT2 inhibitors for diabetes may result in a serious condition of too much acid in the blood. 2015. Available at: https://www.fda.gov/Drugs/DrugSafety/ucm475463.htm. Accessed May 21, 2019.

21. Ueda P, Svanstrom H, Melbye M, et al. Sodium glucose cotransporter 2 inhibitors and risk of serious adverse events: nationwide register based cohort study. BMJ 2018;363:k4365.

22. Fralick M, Schneeweiss S, Patorno E. risk of diabetic ketoacidosis after initiation of an SGLT2 inhibitor. N Engl J Med 2017;376:2300–2.

23. Zhang X-L, Zhu Q-Q, Chen Y-H. Cardiovascular safety, long-term noncardiovascular safety, and efficacy of sodium-glucose cotransporter 2 inhibitors in patients with type 2 diabetes mellitus: a systemic review and meta-analysis with trial sequential analysis. J Am Heart Assoc 2018;7(2):e007165.

24. Musso G, Gambino R, Cassader M, et al. Efficacy and safety of dual SGLT1/2 inhibitor sotagliflozin in type 1 diabetes: meta-analysis of randomized controlled trials. BMJ 2019;365:11328.

25. Kitabchi AE, Nyenwe EA. Hyperglycemic crises in diabetes mellitus: diabetic ketoacidosis and hyperglycemic hyperosmolar state. Endocrinol Metab Clin North Am 2006;35:725–51.

26. Kitabchi AE, Umpierrez GE, Miles JM, et al. Hyperglycemic crises in adult patients with diabetes. Diabetes Care 2009;32:1335–43.

27. Weinstock RS, Xing D, Maahs DM, et al. Severe hypoglycemia and diabetic ketoacidosis in adults with type 1 diabetes: results from the T1D Exchange Clinic Registry. J Clin Endocrinol Metab 2013;98:3411–9.

28. Akturk HK, Taylor DD, Camsari UM. Association between cannabis use and risk for diabetic ketoacidosis in adults with type 1 diabetes. JAMA Intern Med 2019; 179:115–8.

29. Umpierrez G, Freire AX. Abdominal pain in patients with hyperglycemic crises. J Crit Care 2002;17:63–7.
30. Edge JA, Hawkins MM, Winter DL, et al. The risk and outcome of cerebral oedema developing during diabetic ketoacidosis. Arch Dis Child 2001;85:16–22.
31. Dunger DB, Sperling MA, Acerini CL, et al. ESPE/LWPES consensus statement on diabetic ketoacidosis in children and adolescents. Arch Dis Child 2004;89: 188–94.
32. Lawrence SE, Cummings EA, Gaboury I, et al. Population-based study of incidence and risk factors for cerebral edema in pediatric diabetic ketoacidosis. J Pediatr 2005;146:688–92.
33. Glaser N. Cerebral injury (cerebral edema) in children with diabetic ketoacidosis. Hoppin AG, editor. UpToDate. Waltham (MA): UpToDate Inc. Available at: https://www.uptodate.com. Accessed May 21, 2019.
34. Hirsch IB, Emmett M. Diabetic ketoacidosis and hyperosmolar hyperglycemic state in adults: clinical features, evaluation, and diagnosis. Nathan DM, editor. UpToDate. Waltham (MA): UpToDate Inc. Available at: https://www.uptodate.com. Accessed February 12, 2019.
35. Nair S, Yadav D, Pitchumoni CS. Association of diabetic ketoacidosis and acute pancreatitis: observations in 100 consecutive episodes of DKA. Am J Gastroenterol 2000;95:2795–800.
36. Brutsaert EF. Diabetic ketoacidosis. In: Porter RS, Kaplan JL, editors. Merck manual professional version. Whitehouse Station (NJ): Merck Sharp & Dohme Corp; 2018. Subscription required to view. Available at: http://online.statref.com. Accessed February 12, 2019.
37. Wilson HK, Keuer SP, Lea AS. Phosphate therapy in diabetic ketoacidosis. Arch Intern Med 1982;142:517–20.
38. Firestone RL, Parker PL, Pandya KA, et al. Moderate-intensity insulin therapy is associated with reduced length of stay in critically ill patients with diabetic ketoacidosis and hyperosmolar hyperglycemic state. Crit Care Med 2019;47:700–5.
39. Kraut J, Madias NE. Treatment of acute metabolic acidosis: a pathophysiologic approach. Nat Rev Nephrol 2012;8:589–601.
40. Nugent BW. Hyperosmolar hyperglycemic state. Emerg Med Clin North Am 2005; 23:629–48.
41. Bagdure D, Rewers A, Campagna E, et al. Epidemiology of hyperglycemic hyperosmolar syndrome in children hospitalized in USA. Pediatr Diabetes 2013;14: 18–24.
42. Agrawal S, Baird GL, Quintos JB, et al. Pediatric diabetic ketoacidosis with hyperosmolarity: clinical characteristics and outcomes. Endocr Pract 2018;24:726–32.
43. Bhansali A, Sukumar SP. Hyperosmolar hyperglycemic state. In: Mohan V, Umnikrishnan R, editors. World clinics diabetology: complications of diabetesvol. 2. New Delhi (India): Jaypee Brothers Medical Publishers, Ltd; 2016. p. 1–10.
44. Trence DL, Hirsch IB. Hyperglycemic crises in diabetes mellitus type 2. Endocrinol Metab Clin North Am 2001;30:817–31.
45. American Diabetes Association. Standards of medical care in diabetes. Diabetes Care 2018;41(Suppl 1):S1–159 (Table 6.3).
46. Seaquist ER, Anderson J, Childs B, et al. Hypoglycemia and diabetes: a report of a workshop of the American Diabetes Association and the Endocrine Society. Diabetes Care 2013;36:1384–95.
47. Spanakis EK, Cryer PE, Davis SN. Hypoglycemia during therapy of diabetes. In: Feingold KR, Anawalt B, Boyce A, et al, editors. Endotext - NCBI bookshelf. South

Dartmouth (MA): MDText.com, Inc; 2018. Available at: http://www.endotext.org. Accessed February 12, 2019.

48. Elliott L, Fidler C, Ditchfield A, et al. Hypoglycemia event rates: a comparison between real-world data and randomized controlled trial populations in insulin-treated diabetes. Diabetes Ther 2016;7:45–60.

49. Strachan MWJ. Frequency, causes and risk factors for hypoglycaemia in type 1 diabetes. In: Frier BM, Heller SR, McCrimmon RJ, editors. Hypoglycaemia in clinical diabetes. 3rd edition. Chichester (United Kingdom): Wiley-Blackwell; 2014. p. 63–95.

50. Khunti K, Alsifri s, Aronson M, et al. Rates and predictors of hypoglycemia in 27,585 people from 24 countries with insulin-treated type 1 and type 2 diabetes: the global HAT study. Diabetes Obes Metab 2016;18:907–15.

51. Pedersen-Bjergaard U, Thorsteinsson B. Reporting severe hypoglycemia in type 1 diabetes: facts and pitfalls. Curr Diab Rep 2017;17:131.

52. Lamounier RN, Geloneze B, Leite SO, et al. Hypoglycemia incidence and awareness among insulin-treated patients with diabetes: the HAT study in Brazil. Diabetol Metab Syndr 2018;10:83.

53. McCoy RG, Van Houten HK, Ziegenfuss JY, et al. Self-report of hypoglycemia and health-related quality of life in patients with type 1 and type 2 diabetes. Endocr Pract 2013;19:792–9.

54. Cryer PE. Hypoglycemia in type 1 diabetes mellitus. Endocrinol Metab Clin North Am 2010;39:641–54.

55. McCoy RG, Van Houten HK, Ziegenfuss JY, et al. Increased mortality of patients with diabetes reporting severe hypoglycemia. Diabetes Care 2012;35:1897–901.

56. Cryer PE. Glycemic goals in diabetes: trade-off between glycemic control and iatrogenic hypoglycemia. Diabetes 2014;63:2188–95.

57. Cryer PE. Mechanisms of hypoglycemia-associated autonomic failure and its component syndromes in diabetes. Diabetes 2005;54:3592–601.

58. Zhou M, Wang SV, Leonard CE, et al. Sentinel modular program for propensity score-matched cohort analyses. Application to glyburide, glipizide, and serious hypoglycemia. Epidemiology 2017;28:838–46.

59. Matthew P. Hypoglycemia. In: Thoppil D, editor. StatPearls [Internet]. Treasure Island (FL): StatPearls Publishing; 2018. Available at: https://www.statpearls.com/as/endocrine%20and%20metabolic/23267. Accessed May 21, 2019.

60. Cryer PE. Mechanisms of hypoglycemia-associated autonomic failure in diabetes. N Engl J Med 2013;369:362–72.

61. Beck RW, Bergenstal RM, Riddlesworth TD, et al. The association of biochemical hypoglycemia with the subsequent risk of a severe hypoglycemic event: analysis of the DCCT data set. Diabetes Technol Ther 2019;21:1–5.

62. Saydah S, Imperatore G, Divers J, et al. Occurrence of severe hypoglycaemic events among US youth and young adults with type 1 and type 2 diabetes. Endocrinol Diabetes Metab 2019;2:e00057.

63. Henriksen MM, Andersen HU, Thorsteinsson B, et al. Hypoglycemic exposure and risk of asymptomatic hypoglycemia in type 1 diabetes assessed by continuous glucose monitoring. Endocrinol Metab 2018;103:2329–35.

64. Lipska KJ, Warton EM, Moffet HH, et al. HbA1c and risk of severe hypoglycemia in type 2 diabetes. Diabetes Care 2013;36:3535–42.

65. Geelhoed-Duijvestijn PH, Pedersen-Bjergaard U, Weitgasser R, et al. Effects of patient-reported non-severe hypoglycemia on healthcare resource use, work-time loss, and wellbeing in insulin-treated patients with diabetes in seven European countries. J Med Econ 2013;16:1453–61.

66. Arnaud M, Pariente A, Bezin J, et al. Risk of serious trauma with glucose-lowering drugs in older persons: a nested case-control study. J Am Geriatr Soc 2018;66: 2086–91.
67. Cryer PE. Hypoglycemia in adults with diabetes mellitus. In: Hirsch IB, Mulder JE, editors. UpToDate. Waltham (MA): UpToDate Inc. Available at: https://www.uptodate.com. Accessed February 12, 2019.
68. Rickels MR, Ruedy KJ, Foster NC, et al. Intranasal glucagon for treatment of insulin-induced hypoglycemia in adults with type 1 diabetes: a randomized crossover noninferiority study. Diabetes Care 2016;39:264–70.
69. Haymond MW, DuBose SN, Rickels MR, et al. Efficacy and safety of mini-dose glucagon for treatment of nonsevere hypoglycemia in adults with type 1 diabetes. J Clin Endocrinol Metab 2017;102:2994–3001.
70. Irvine AA, Cox D, Gonder-Frederick L. Fear of hypoglycemia: relationship to physical and psychological symptoms in patients with insulin-dependent diabetes mellitus. Health Psychol 1992;11:135–8.
71. Yeo E, Choudhary P, Nwokolo M, et al. Interventions that restore awareness of hypoglycemia in adults with type 1 diabetes: a systematic review and meta-analysis. Diabetes Care 2015;38:1592–609.
72. Beck RW, Riddlesworth TD, Ruedy K, et al. Continuous glucose monitoring versus usual care in patients with type 2 diabetes receiving multiple daily insulin injections: a randomized trial. Ann Intern Med 2017;16:365–74.

Living Day to Day
Chronic Complications

Gerald Kayingo, PhD, MMSc, PA-C*,
Virginia McCoy Hass, RN, DNP, FNP-C, PA-C

KEYWORDS

- Diabetes • Chronic complications • Micro and macro vascular disease
- Retinopathy • Neuropathy • Nephropathy • Depression
- Coordinated and patient-centered care

KEY POINTS

- Diabetes is a complex chronic disease causing multiple complications that involve almost all body systems. These complications are the result of both microvascular and macrovascular changes.
- Complications of diabetes also include dermopathy, infection, lower extremity amputation, periodontal disease, sexual and bladder dysfunction, and depression.
- Glycemic control and routine health maintenance are key in preventing and reducing complications associated with diabetes. Patient-centered team-based care improves outcomes and should be accessible to all patients with diabetes.
- At office or clinic visits, clinicians should perform a comprehensive history and physical examination to assess for manifestations of diabetes complications.
- Early diagnosis of complications is critical in preventing the disease progression.

INTRODUCTION

The worldwide prevalence of diabetes (DM) is rising (**Box 1**). Type I DM (T1DM) is characterized by dependence on exogenous insulin, whereas type II DM (T2DM) is characterized by relative insulin deficiency and/or resistance.[5] As of 2018, there were estimated to be more than 500 million patients with DM, of whom 90% had T2DM.[6,7] In the United States, DM affects more than 29 million people and the prevalence is increasing.[8,9] Patients with DM may develop multiple chronic complications that can involve almost all body systems (**Fig. 1**). DM-related complications can be grouped into vascular and nonvascular complications. The vascular complications are further divided into macrovascular (coronary artery disease, peripheral arterial

Betty Irene Moore School of Nursing, University of California, Davis, Administrative Support Building, 2450 48th Street Suite 2120, Sacramento, CA 95817, USA
* Corresponding author.
E-mail address: gkayingo@ucdavis.edu

Physician Assist Clin 5 (2020) 213–224
https://doi.org/10.1016/j.cpha.2019.12.002
2405-7991/20/© 2019 Elsevier Inc. All rights reserved.

physicianassistant.theclinics.com

Box 1
Chronic Care Model (CCM)[1] for managing diabetes and the associated complications

The chronic care model (CCM) has been shown to be effective approach in managing diabetes and the associated complications.[1-4] The CCM has 6 core elements that ensure optimal care of patients with chronic diseases.

- The community
  - Advocate for community policies and resources needed for chronic care

- The healthy system
  - Create a culture of patient safety, high-quality care

- Self-management support
  - Empower patients to manage their health and care
  - Enable self-management action plans

- Delivery system design
  - Incorporate cultural competency and health literacy concepts
  - Facilitate case management

- Decision support
  - Provide clinical care that is consistent with scientific evidence
  - Use evidence-based practices

- Clinical information systems
  - Use patient- and population-level data when offering care
  - Implement care coordination and patient registries

---

disease, and stroke) or microvascular complications (diabetic retinopathy, nephropathy, and neuropathy) (**Box 2**).

PATHOPHYSIOLOGY OF COMPLICATIONS OF DIABETES

The pathophysiology and pathogenesis of DM-induced vascular damage involve multiple metabolic pathways including the polyol pathway, advanced glycation end products (AGEs) accumulation, defective stimulation of phosphatidylinositol 3-kinase activity, the protein kinase C pathway, and the hexosamine pathway.[10-12] Studies have demonstrated that these mechanisms are common to both microvascular and macrovascular complications (see **Fig. 1**). Nonvascular complications of DM include fatty liver, cataract, and diabetic dermopathy.[13] Additionally, several recent studies and meta-analyses have identified increased risk for specific types of cancer in patients with DM including liver, pancreas, colorectal, kidney, bladder, endometrial, and breast cancers, as well as non-Hodgkin's lymphoma.[13] The evidence for increased risk is greatest for malignancies of the liver (relative risk, 2.51; 95% confidence interval, 1.9–3.2) and the pancreas (relative risk, 1.94; 95% confidence interval, 1.53–2.46).[14] The etiology of increased incidence of malignancy in patients with DM is hypothesized as both general mechanisms (hyperinsulinemia, hyperglycemia, and obesity) and organ-specific factors; however, the exact mechanisms are not yet understood.

OPHTHALMIC COMPLICATIONS OF DIABETES

Worldwide, retinopathy is the most common microvascular complication of DM and is the most common cause of blindness for working-age adults in developed countries.[11,15] The risk of retinopathy increases with duration of DM and is directly correlated to poor glycemic control, the presence of albuminuria, and elevated diastolic blood pressure.[16] In addition, the hormonal and immunologic changes of pregnancy are independent risk factors for the onset or progression of diabetic retinopathy.[15]

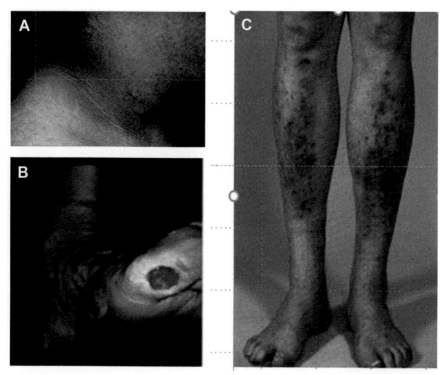

Fig. 1. Dermatologic manifestations of diabetes. (*A*) Acanthosis nigricans. (*B*) Diabetic foot ulcers. (*D*) Diabetic dermopathy.

There are 2 types of diabetic retinopathy: nonproliferative diabetic retinopathy (NPDR) and proliferative diabetic retinopathy (PDR). The clinical features of NPDR include venous dilation, microaneurysms, retinal hemorrhages, retinal edema, cotton wool spots, venous beading, and hard exudates. PDR develops in response to the chronic retinal hypoxia that develops as NPDR progresses. PDR is characterized by neovascularization (formation of new retinal blood vessels). These new vessels are weak, resulting in vitreous hemorrhages and an increased risk of sudden and severe vision loss. PDR is found more commonly in T1DM and diabetic macular edema (DME) is more common in T2DM.[17]

DME is the leading cause of moderate to severe vision loss in this population. It is defined as retinal thickening or the presence of hard exudates in or adjacent to the macula.[17] DME is found in both NPDR and PDR and occurs independent of the severity of the retinopathy.[17]

Additional ophthalmic complications of DM include cataracts and glaucoma. Patients with DM have up to a 5-fold greater risk for cataract formation, with earlier age at onset as compared with the nondiabetic population. AGEs, the polyol pathway, and increased oxidative stress are proposed mechanisms.[17]

DM is the primary cause of neovascular glaucoma, which is an intractable type of glaucoma. Neovascular glaucoma is most commonly seen in conjunction with PDR, but can occur in patients without preexisting neovascularization. Glaucoma may also be a secondary complication of the treatment of other diabetic ocular diseases, for example, after laser panretinal photocoagulation for the treatment of PDR.[17]

Box 2
Chronic complications of diabetes

Microvascular

- Eye diseases
- Retinopathy (proliferative and nonproliferative)
- Macular edema
- Peripheral neuropathy
- Sensory neuropathy
- Motor (mononeuropathy and polyneuropathy)
- Autonomic neuropathy
  - Gastrointestinal complications such has gastroparesis, constipation, and diarrhea
  - Genitourinary complications including uropathy and sexual dysfunction
  - Cardiac autonomic neuropathy
- Nephropathy
- Albuminuria
- Declining kidney function, chronic kidney disease, end-stage renal disease

Macrovascular

- Coronary heart disease
- Peripheral arterial disease
- Cerebrovascular disease

Other complications

- Dermatologic
  - Diabetic dermopathy
  - Diabetic ulcers
  - Acanthosis nigricans
  - Infections (bacterial and fungal)
  - Diabetic cheiroarthropathy
- Ocular
  - Cataracts
  - Glaucoma
- Periodontal disease
- Hearing loss
- Cognitive impairment/dementia

Because early diabetic retinopathy is asymptomatic without pain or vision loss, screening guidelines for diabetic retinopathy include annual dilated eye examinations for all patients with DM. Ophthalmic examinations should be performed beginning at age 11 or 5 years after the diagnosis of T1DM (whichever is earlier) and at the time of diagnosis of T2DM.[15] Patients with preexisting DM who present with new vision changes should have a retinal examination within 1 to 3 days.[15] Guidelines offer direction for ocular evaluation during pregnancy.[18] Women with preexisting DM who are planning to become pregnant should have retinopathy screening before conception. Women with preexisting DM who become pregnant and have not had a retinal examination within the last 12 months should be referred for screening at their first prenatal appointment. If retinopathy is found at preconception or early pregnancy screening, referral should be guided by standards of care and the woman should be evaluated by an ophthalmologist within 4 weeks. If any retinopathy is found at the initial prenatal visit, an additional assessment should be made at 16 to 20 weeks of gestation or as determined by the ophthalmologist. If no retinopathy is found at the initial prenatal visit, an additional screening should be made at 28 weeks of gestation.[18] **Box 3** outlines the recommended timing of retinal examinations in patients with DM.

Key strategies for the prevention and treatment of ocular complications in patients with DM include optimizing glycemic and blood pressure control, and management of hyperlipidemia. Effective treatment, such as laser photocoagulation, is available for both severe DME and early PDR if diabetic retinopathy is recognized early. Moderate to severe PDR must be treated with vitreoretinal surgery. The prognosis for preservation of vision is less optimistic even with therapy. Anti-vascular endothelial growth factor (anti-VEGF) therapy offers remarkable clinical benefits for patients with severe macular edema involving the fovea.[15] Anti-VEGF medication is injected directly into the vitreous, allowing for a high local concentration and minimized systemic side effects. Anti-VEGF therapy requires multiple injections and carries a small risk of systemic thrombosis and ocular infection.[15] Intravitreal sustained release steroid implants are also used for chronic DME. These offer additional anti-inflammatory effects as compared with anti-VEGF injection. Like anti-VEGF therapy, intraocular steroid implants also carry the risk of postoperative infection. Additionally, there is a risk of steroid-induced cataract and/or glaucoma.[15]

KIDNEY COMPLICATIONS OF DIABETES (NEPHROPATHY)

DM is the most common cause of chronic kidney disease (CKD) worldwide.[19] The prevalence of nephropathy, evidenced by albuminuria, varies widely by DM type, ranging from 15% to 40% in patients with T1DM to 5% to 20% in patients with T2DM.[11]

There is a strong association between diabetic retinopathy and diabetic nephropathy; the underlying pathophysiologic mechanisms are the same: oxidative stress, accumulation of AGEs, and activation of intracellular signaling molecules such as protein kinase C.[11] DM induces changes in the microvasculature of the capillary basement membrane, including the arterioles of the glomeruli. The resulting increase in capillary permeability results in albuminuria, the hallmark of diabetic nephropathy.[11,19]

Box 3	
Recommended timing of retinal examination for patients with diabetes	
Patient Characteristics	**Timing of Retinal Examination**
Initial diagnosis of T2DM	At age 11 or 5 y after diagnosis (whichever is first)
Initial diagnosis of T1DM	At time of diagnosis
No diabetic retinopathy	Annually
Presence of diabetic retinopathy	Based on the severity of retinopathy (eg, every 3–6 mo)
Presence of visual symptoms	Within 1–3 d
Loss of vision	Preconception
New reading difficulties	At first prenatal visit if no done within prior 12 mo
Altered color perception	Reassess at 16–20 weeks of gestation if any retinopathy at initial screen
New moving dark spots	Reassess at 28 weeks of gestation if no retinopathy at initial screen
Women planning pregnancy	
Women who are pregnant	

Data from Nentwich, M. M., & Ulbig, M. W. (2015). Diabetic retinopathy - ocular complications of diabetes mellitus. World Journal of Diabetes, 6(3), 489- 499.

The degree of albuminuria is both indicative of the severity of nephropathy and the risk for progression to CKD. CKD is defined as the persistence for longer than 3 months of markers of kidney damage *or* decline in glomerular filtration rate (**Box 4**).[11] As of 2017, the incidence of end-stage renal disease leading to dialysis, transplantation, or death was 124,500 new cases, with a prevalence of 746,557 cases in the United States with an increase of 20,000 cases per year.[20] This reflects a continued upward trend from 2012 to 2016 attributed to the aging US population and the increased prevalence of obesity and DM in the general population.[20] To decrease the prevalence of diabetic nephropathy, the Kidney Disease Improving Global Outcomes CKD Work Group guideline recommends the following[19]:

- Using both a spot urine sample for urine albumin:creatine ratio and a glomerular filtration rate
  - Screen all patients with T2DM at initial diagnosis, then annually
  - Screen all patients with T1DM 5 years after initial diagnosis, then annually
- Screen all patients for comorbid hypertension

Therapy directed at decreasing urinary albumin excretion rate may slow the progression of diabetic nephropathy. Angiotensin-converting enzyme inhibitors and angiotensin receptor blockers (ARB) have been shown to reduce urinary albumin excretion rate, even if comorbid hypertension is not present.[19] Treatment with an angiotensin-converting enzyme inhibitors or ARB is recommended for patients with DM and hypertension and for patients with DM, normotension and albuminuria (defined as an albumin:creatinine ratio of $\geq$30 mg/dL[20]) who are at high risk of nephropathy or its progression, it is to be considered.[19] Initiation of angiotensin-converting enzyme inhibitor/ARB treatment starts at a low dose with titration up to maximum doses for hypertension management. When starting these medications, one must monitor the serum creatinine and potassium levels. The goal is to titrate therapies to normalize urine albumin excretion to less than 30 mg/g on at least 2 of 3 urine samples checked every 6 months.[19] Recently, treatment with canagliflozin (Invokana), a sodium-glucose cotransporter 2 inhibitor was shown to decrease progression to end-stage renal disease when initiated in patients with T2DM and greater than 300 mg/dL albuminuria. A team-based approach should be used to optimize glycemic and blood pressure control.

Box 4
Criteria for the diagnosis of CKD

Markers of Kidney Damage	Decline in the GFR
Persistence for $\geq$3 mo of either: Albuminuria ($\geq$30 mg/24 h; albumin:creatinine ratio of $\geq$30 mg/g) Urine sediment abnormalities Electrolyte and other abnormalities owing to tubular disorders Renal abnormalities detected by histology Structural renal anomalies on imaging History of kidney transplantation	GFR <60 mL/min/1.73 m^2 (GFR categories G3a–G5)

Abbreviation: GFR, glomerular filtration rate.

Data from KDIGO. Kidney Disease: Improving Global Outcomes (KDIGO) CKD Work Group (2013). KDIGO 2012 Clinical Practice Guideline for the Evaluation and Management of Chronic Kidney Disease. In: *Kidney International*;pp. 1-150.

NEUROLOGIC COMPLICATIONS OF DIABETES (NEUROPATHY)

Peripheral or autonomic neuropathy affects nearly 50% of patients with DM.[11] Neuropathy is a microvascular complication of DM via multifactorial mechanisms that are, as yet, poorly understood.[21] Clinical signs and symptoms may include pain, tingling, numbness, and/or buzzing sensations in hands and/or feet. Autonomic manifestations of neuropathy may include poor bladder control, gastroparesis, constipation, loss of balance and/or sexual dysfunction. Cardiac autonomic neuropathy may result in silent ischemia, orthostatic hypotension, and cardiac dysrhythmia.[22] Patients with peripheral neuropathy are at increased risk for extremity injuries, infection, ulcers and lower extremity amputation.

As with other complication of DM, glycemic control and management of cardiovascular risk factors are the cornerstones of prevention. Patients should perform self-foot examinations daily, but the practitioner foot examination is vitally important. Not only do patients with DM have decreased sensitivity, they often have decreased vision and are unable to examine the bottom of their feet. Thus, the practitioner is often the person to see a foot issue first and is able to intervene before a loss of a limb. In fact, because of the importance of the foot examination, Medicare pays for podiatric care.[23]

CARDIOVASCULAR COMPLICATIONS OF DIABETES

T2DM commonly occurs in the context of metabolic syndrome (abdominal obesity, hyperglycemia, hypertension, hyperlipidemia, and increased coagulability). This comorbid constellation of disorders works synergistically to cause atherosclerosis and increase the risk of cardiovascular disease (see **Fig. 1**). Atherosclerotic cardiovascular disease can occur in any artery and results in coronary artery disease, peripheral arterial disease, and/or cerebrovascular disease (stroke) depending on the site. Overlap of these cardiovascular diseases is common and the presence of one should prompt investigation for the others.[24]

In addition to close glycemic control, recommendations for primary prevention of atherosclerotic cardiovascular disease in patients with DM include

1. Risk stratification and treatment guided by calculation of the 10-year atherosclerotic cardiovascular disease risk using the American College of Cardiology/American Heart Association risk calculator (http://tools.acc.org/ASCVD-Risk-Estimator-Plus/#!/calculate/estimate/)
2. Screening for hypertension at every clinical visit
3. Individualization of blood pressure targets based on comorbid conditions
4. Guideline-directed pharmacologic management of hypertension to include an angiotensin-converting enzyme inhibitors or ARB at the maximum tolerated dose as first-line treatment in patients with DM and an albumin:creatinine ratio of $\geq$30 mg/g[25]
5. Guideline-directed lipid lowering therapy with a statin[26]
6. Lifestyle interventions: weight loss if appropriate, Dietary Approaches to Stop Hypertension or Mediterranean diet, moderation of alcohol intake, and increased physical activity[27] (**Box 5**).

In general, the following considerations should be taken when choosing hypoglycemic agent in the pharmacologic management of T2DM:

- Avoid thiazolidinediones (TZD) in patients with heart failure or significant peripheral edema as this drug class can increase fluid retention.
- Discontinue metformin in the setting of
  - GFR <30 ml/min
  - Unstable heart failure
  - Shock

Box 5
Strategies to reduce the risk of complications from DM

Glucose control
- Check hemoglobin A1C every 3 to 6 months
- Goal hemoglobin A1C of less than 7% depending on comorbidities and age

Blood pressure control
- Measure blood pressure every visit
- Maintain blood pressure levels of less than 130/80 mm Hg[11]

Lipids
- Encourage lipid lowering drugs (statins) because they aid in decreasing atherosclerotic cardiovascular disease events associated with DM.
- Lipid-lowering therapy is recommended for:
  o Patients with DM (40–75 years of age) with LDL-C levels of greater than 70 mg/dL

Kidney function
- Check serum creatinine and urinary albumin-to-creatinine ratio annually

Smoking cessation
- Discontinuation of smoking reduces risk of complications and increases survival[10]

Aspirin
- Recommend aspirin (75–162 mg/d) for secondary prevention of cardiovascular disease[12]
- Recommend aspirin (75–162 mg/d) for primary prevention in patients with DM at increased cardiovascular risk (10-year risk of >10%)

Medications
- Offer angiotensin-converting enzyme inhibitory therapy

Immunizations, vaccinations, and routine health maintenance
- To reduce the risk of infections and associated complications, patients with DM should
  o Receive annual influenza vaccinations
  o Receive a tetanus booster every 10 years
  o Zoster vaccine
  o Get pneumococcal vaccine once as an adult before 65 years of age and then 2 more doses at 65 years or older
  o Get the hepatitis vaccine if unvaccinated adults and younger than 60 years of age
- For routine health monitoring, patients with DM should receive
  o Annual dilated eye examination
  o Annual comprehensive foot examination
  o Annual dental examination
- Routine dietary and exercise counseling

SKIN COMPLICATIONS ASSOCIATED WITH DIABETES

Skin disorders of people with DM frequently precede the diagnosis of DM and may be important for its initial identification. Patients with DM experience a variety of skin conditions, including infections, itching, ulcers, and pigmentation changes. In most cases, the underlying pathophysiology is chronic hyperglycemia, hyperinsulinemia, and associated impaired immunity. Hyperglycemia alters keratinocyte function, vasodilation, and produces direct cellular damage through AGEs and proinflammatory cytokines.[28] Additionally, diabetic polyneuropathy and micrangiopathy play important roles in the development of skin complications of this disease. Polyneuropathy and correlated dysfunction of sweating owing to impairment of the sympathetic nerve system may result in subclinical xerosis and diabetic pruritus.[28]

Dermopathy presents with brown atrophic macules and patches on the legs; often precipitated by trauma. Acanthosis nigricans manifests as velvety, brown, hyperpigmented plaques around the neck, axillae, and other flexural surfaces.[28] Patients with DM are susceptible to bacterial skin infections such as styes, folliculitis, carbuncles, and paronychia. The most common organisms include *Staphylococcus aureus*, *Streptococcus pneumoniae*, and *Pseudomonas spp*. Physical examination of the infected skin yields variable symptoms based on the infectious agent and, in severe cases, systemic symptoms such as malaise, fever, and chills may be present. In addition to bacterial infections, fungal skin infections are common, often with *Candida albicans*. Recurrent yeast infections (eg, vaginal, intertriginous, foot) should trigger further investigation for previously undiagnosed DM.

OTHER CHRONIC COMPLICATIONS OF DIABETES

An overview of chronic complications of DM is shown in **Box 2**. DM affects the whole gastrointestinal tract with presenting symptoms of esophageal dysmotility, gastroparesis, constipation, diarrhea, and/or fecal incontinence. Often these chronic gastrointestinal symptoms are very disruptive to the patient and work to isolate the patient from friends and family and can lead to psychosocial distress.[29] Practitioners should suspect gastroparesis if patients present with erratic glucose control or with upper gastrointestinal symptoms without another identified cause. Gastroparesis should be managed by optimizing glycemic control and concentrating on a low-fat/low-fiber diet. A referral to a dietician is appropriate and covered by most insurance policies.

In 1998, Bob Dole, war hero, Kansas congressman, and Republican presidential candidate, announced to the world that he had erectile dysfunction. Suddenly, the never talked about condition associated with aging became a common conversation topic. Advertisements for products, both legitimate and not so legitimate, appeared on television, in magazines, and were displayed in pharmacies, gas stations, and what seemed like everywhere. And a whole new aspect of living with DM came to the forefront: sexual dysfunction. Neuropathy, commonly associated with DM, is a factor in erectile dysfunction. It is more common in those with poor blood sugar control and/or those with a longer duration of DM.[30]

Because of the neurogenic effects on the urinary system, bladder dysfunction, dyspareunia, and retrograde ejaculation are also more common in patients with DM.[31] Estimates are that up to 20% of men with DMT1 and 38% of women experience lower urinary tract symptoms.[32]

The National Institute of Diabetes and Digestive and Kidney Diseases devotes an entire section to sexual and bladder problems along with foot problems, eye diseases, neuropathy, and dental and cardiovascular involvement.

Other conditions more common in male patients with DM include retrograde ejaculation, Peyronie's disease, and low testosterone levels. Women have more instance of cystitis and vaginal yeast. Both genders can experience decreased libido and fertility.

SUMMARY

Patients with DM are more prone to both microvascular and macrovascular chronic complications. These complications include but are not limited to diabetic retinopathy, neuropathy, and nephropathy, along with cardiovascular complications. Outcomes of poorly controlled DM can include myocardial infarctions, blindness, kidney failure, peripheral article disease, stroke, and amputations, as well as other complications. The clinical manifestations of microvascular and macrovascular complications are highly variable in the patient with diabetes. Early recognition and good glucose control are vital to prevent or reduce complications. Practitioners should perform a comprehensive history and physical examination checking for systemic manifestations of DM. Timely screenings, therapies, and referrals (cardiology, podiatry, and ophthalmology, among others) should be offered to all patients with DM. Highlighting the chronic issues that can occur with DM during appointments for routine health maintenance is important for the patient with DM. A patient-centered team-based chronic care model is known to improve outcomes.[1–3]

Managing chronic complications should be follow a team-based care philosophy. A systemic, proactive, patient-centered, and evidence-based approach improves outcomes and leads to healthier lives in patients with DM and the associated chronic complications.

DISCLOSURE

Nothing to disclose.

REFERENCES

1. Stellefson M, Dipnarine K, Stopka C. The chronic care model and diabetes management in US primary care settings: a systematic review. Prev Chronic Dis 2013; 10:E26.
2. Bodenheimer T, Wagner EH, Grumbach K. Improving primary care for patients with chronic illness. JAMA 2002;288(14):1775–9.
3. Bodenheimer T, Wagner EH, Grumbach K. Improving primary care for patients with chronic illness: the chronic care model, part 2. JAMA 2002;288(15):1909–14.
4. Hass V, Kayingo G. Chronic care perspectives. In: Ballweg R, Brown D, Vetrosky D, et al, editors. Physician assistant: a guide to clinical practice. 6th edition. Elsevier Health Sciences.
5. Kalofoutis C, Piperi C, Kalofoutis A, et al. Type II diabetes mellitus and cardiovascular risk factors: current therapeutic approaches. Exp Clin Cardiol 2007;12(1): 17–28.
6. You W, Henneberg M. Type 1 diabetes prevalence increasing globally and regionally: the role of natural selection and life expectancy at birth. BMJ Open Diabetes Res Care 2016;4(1):e000161.
7. Kaiser AB, Zhang N, Van der Pluijm W. Global prevalence of type 2 diabetes over the next ten years (2018-2028). Poster session. Diabetes 2018. Available at: https://diabetes.diabetesjournals.org/content/67/Supplement_1/202-LB.
8. Centers for Disease Control and Prevention. Diabetes report card 2014. Atlanta (GA): Centers for Disease Control and Prevention, U.S. Dept of Health and Human Services; 2015. Available at: https://www.cdc.gov/diabetes/pdfs/library/diabetesreportcard2014.pdf. Accessed September, 2019.
9. Raghupathi W, Raghupathi V. An empirical study of chronic diseases in the United States: a visual analytics approach to public health. Int J Environ Res Public Health 2018;15(3):431.
10. Brownlee M. The pathobiology of diabetic complications: a unifying mechanism. Diabetes 2005;54(6):1615–25.
11. Chawla A, Chawla R, Jaggi S. Microvascular and macrovascular complications in diabetes mellitus: distinct or continuum? Indian J Endocrinol Metab 2016;20(4): 546–51.
12. Bouzakri K, Roques M, Gual P, et al. Reduced activation of phosphatidylinositol-3 kinase and increased serine 636 phosphorylation of insulin receptor substrate-1 in primary culture of skeletal muscle cells from patients with type 2 diabetes. Diabetes 2003;52(6):1319–25.

13. Ahmed SS, Laila RT, Thamilselvam P, et al. Knowledge of risk factors and compli-
    cations of diabetes in the Indian ethnic population of Malaysia undiagnosed to
    have diabetes. Int J Diabetes Res 2019;8(1):4–8.
14. Vigneri P, Frasca F, Sciacca L, et al. Diabetes and cancer. Endocr Relat Cancer
    2009;16(4):1103–23.
15. Nentwich MM, Ulbig MW. Diabetic retinopathy - ocular complications of diabetes
    mellitus. World J Diabetes 2015;6(3):489–99.
16. Hainsworth DP, Bebu I, Aiello LP, et al, for the Diabetes Control and Complica-
    tions Trial (DCCT)/Epidemiology of Diabetes Interventions and Complications
    (EDIC) Research Group. Risk factors for retinopathy in type 1 diabetes: the
    DCCT/EDIC study. Diabetes Care 2019;42(5):875–82.
17. Sayin N, Kara N, Pekel G. Ocular complications of diabetes mellitus. World J Dia-
    betes 2015;6(1):92–108.
18. National Collaborating Centre for Women's and Children's Health (UK). Diabetes
    in pregnancy: management of diabetes and its complications from preconcep-
    tion to the postnatal period. London: National Institute for Health and Care Excel-
    lence (UK); 2015.
19. Levin A, Stevens PE, Bilous RW, et al. Kidney Disease: Improving Global Out-
    comes (KDIGO) CKD Work Group. KDIGO 2012 clinical practice guideline for
    the evaluation and management of chronic kidney disease. Kidney International
    Supplements 2013;3(1):1–150.
20. United States Renal Data System. 2019 USRDS annual data report: epidemiology
    of kidney disease in the United States. Bethesda (MD): National Institutes of
    Health, National Institute of Diabetes and Digestive and Kidney Diseases; 2019.
21. Watterworth B, Wright TB. Diabetic peripheral neuropathy. In: Abd-Elsayed A, ed-
    itor. Pain. Cham (Switzerland): Springer; 2019. p. 911–3.
22. Spallone V. Update on the impact, diagnosis and management of cardiovascular
    autonomic neuropathy in diabetes: what is defined, what is new, and what is un-
    met. Diabetes Metab J 2019;43(1):3–30.
23. Centers for Medicare and Medicaid Services. Foot care. Available at: https://
    www.medicare.gov/coverage/foot-care. Accessed August 30, 2019.
24. Alberts MJ, Bhatt DL, Mas JL, et al, for the REduction of Atherothrombosis for
    Continued Health Registry Investigators. Three-year follow-up and event rates
    in the international REduction of Atherothrombosis for Continued Health Registry.
    Eur Heart J 2009;30(19):2318–26.
25. Whelton PK, Carey RM, Aronow WS, et al. ACC/AHA/AAPA/ABC/ACPM/AGS/
    APhA/ASH/ASPC/NMA/PCNA guideline for the prevention, detection, evaluation,
    and management of high blood pressure in adults: a report of the American Col-
    lege of Cardiology/American Heart Association Task Force on Clinical Practice
    Guidelines. J Am Coll Cardiol 2018;71:e127–248.
26. Arnett DK, Khera A, Blumenthal RS. 2019 ACC/AHA guideline on the primary pre-
    vention of cardiovascular disease. JAMA Cardiol 2019;4(10):1043–4.
27. American Diabetes Association. The 2019 standards of medical care in diabetes.
    Diabetes Care 2019;42(Supplement 1):S103–23.
28. Lima AL, Illing T, Schliemann S, et al. Cutaneous manifestations of diabetes mel-
    litus: a review. Am J Clin Dermatol 2017;18(4):541–53.
29. Du YT, Rayner CK, Jones KL, et al. Gastrointestinal symptoms in diabetes: prev-
    alence, assessment, pathogenesis, and management. Diabet Med 2018;41(3):
    627–37.

30. Kalter-Leibovici O, Wainstein J, Ziv A, et al. Clinical, socioeconomic, and lifestyle parameters associated with erectile dysfunction among diabetic men. Diabetes Care 2005;28:1739.
31. Kempler P, Amarenco G, Freeman R, et al. Management strategies for gastrointestinal, erectile, bladder, and sudomotor dysfunction in patients with diabetes. Diabetes Metab Res Rev 2011;27:665–77.
32. Sarma AV, Kanaya A, Nyberg LM, et al. Risk factors for urinary incontinence among women with type 1 diabetes: findings from the epidemiology of diabetes interventions and complications study. Urology 2009;73:1203–9.

And Baby Makes 2
Gestational Diabetes

Heidi M. Webb, MMS, PA-C, AAPA, ASEPA

KEYWORDS

- Gestational diabetes mellitus (GDM) • Pregnancy complications • GDM screening
- GDM management

KEY POINTS

- Gestational diabetes mellitus (GDM) is a health crisis with increasing prevalence due to the ongoing obesity and type 2 diabetes epidemics. GDM has significant health effects on both the mother and fetus during pregnancy and long term.
- Diagnosis and management of GDM is essential to reduce adverse pregnancy outcomes. Guidelines now support universal screening include screening for high-risk women at initial appointments.
- Treatment for GDM requires a team-based approach. The hallmarks of management of GDM remains lifestyle modification and self-monitoring blood glucose; however, no concrete guidelines exist in regards to nutrition or exercise therapy.

INTRODUCTION

In 1952, Jorgen Pedersen hypothesized that maternal hyperglycemia led to fetal hyperglycemia and an exaggerated response to insulin. The Pedersen hypothesis has formed the groundwork for understanding the pathophysiological consequences of diabetes during pregnancy.[1] Gestational diabetes mellitus (GDM) is defined as glucose intolerance within onset or first recognition during pregnancy, which is distinct from type 1 diabetes mellitus (T1DM) or type 2 diabetes mellitus (T2DM).[1–4] Worldwide incidence has been rising secondary to the obesity and type 2 diabetes epidemics in addition to advancing maternal age.[5,6] The Centers for Disease Control and Prevention (CDC) currently estimates that 2% to 10% of pregnancies annually in the United States are affected by GDM.[2] The exact prevalence is difficult to determine due to lack of universal diagnostic criteria. CDC states that there has been an increase in incidence; before the twenty-first century GDM was found in 3% to 5% of pregnancies.[5] Prevalence can vary widely based on a population's ethnic and racial makeup.[7] The presence of GDM significantly increases the risk of both maternal and fetal complications in the peripartum period and in subsequent years.[6]

Endocrinology and Internal Medicine, Bahl and Bahl Medical Associates, 10922 Frankstown Road, Pittsburgh, PA 15235, USA
E-mail address: heidimwebb@gmail.com

Physician Assist Clin 5 (2020) 225–235
https://doi.org/10.1016/j.cpha.2019.11.008
2405-7991/20/© 2019 Elsevier Inc. All rights reserved.
physicianassistant.theclinics.com

IMPLICATIONS AND RISK—MATERNAL AND FETAL

The 2008 Hyperglycemia and Adverse Pregnancy Outcomes (HAPO) study took a focused look at the associations between adverse outcomes in pregnancy and higher levels of maternal glucose that did not reach diabetic definitions. HAPO sparked discussion and changes regarding criteria for diagnosing GDM and treatment of GDM and established a strong and clear association of increased maternal glucose levels with adverse pregnancy outcomes.[5] GDM has severe implications with both maternal and fetal complications. Even minor disturbances in carbohydrate metabolism are associated with increased morbidity and mortality for both mother and fetus; however, complications are reduced with appropriate management of GDM.[6,8]

Risk of fetal complications in GDM start in utero and may potentially span a lifetime.[9] Fetal complications associated with GDM include an increased risk of macrosomia (birth weight >8 lb 13 oz), shoulder dystocia, neonatal hypoglycemia, and fetal hyperinsulinemia.[7,9] Maternal complications include a high rate of caesarian sections and hypertensive disorders (gestational hypertension, preeclampsia, and eclampsia).[7,9] Congenital abnormalities are not seen with increased frequency in GDM pregnancies because GDM typically occurs later in pregnancy after embryogenesis is complete.[10] Children of women with GDM are at an increased risk of developing obesity, metabolic syndrome, and T2DM at a young age.[7,9] This risk, however, is further affected by environmental factors and genetic susceptibility. Female offspring of women with GDM are also at increased risk of developing GDM.[5,9]

GDM is also associated with increased risk for long-term complications from a maternal standpoint. Women with GDM have a significantly increased risk of development of T2DM. Despite this fact, most women do return to a normoglycemic state after delivery, GDM remains one of the biggest predictive factors for the long-term development of T2DM.[5,7] GDM has been found to also increase the risk of cardiovascular disease (CVD) and metabolic syndrome.[5,7] Eleven and a half years after pregnancy, women with GDM had a 70% higher risk for CVD than matched controls.[7] Women who have had 1 pregnancy with GDM are at increased risk of developing GDM in future pregnancies.[5]

PATHOPHYSIOLOGY

The exact pathophysiology of development of GDM remains unknown. Increased insulin resistance is a normal response to pregnancy.[11] Most theories support insulin resistance and the disruption of pregnancy hormones on the usual action of insulin. Development of GDM typically develops due to β-cell dysfunction on top of a background of insulin resistance.[2,8] GDM is typically associated with obesity; however, it is not limited to overweight or obese women.[8] GDM can also develop in lean women, although the pathway is thought to be different than that seen in overweight or obese women. A small number of women (<10%) have destruction of pancreatic β-cell function as seen in development of T1DM or maturity onset diabetes of the young.[2]

In pregnancy, insulin resistance increases in the late second trimester to levels that approximate those seen in patients with T2DM.[11] In normal pregnancy, a woman must increase insulin secretion by 200% to 250% to maintain a euglycemic state.[5,7] Most women do remain euglycemic due to sufficient β cell compensation. GDM develops if β cell compensation and insulin secretion are inadequate for the level of insulin resistance and hepatic glucose production.[5,11] It is theorized that hormones and adipokines secreted from the placenta, which include tumor necrosis factor alpha (TNF-α), human placental lactogen, and human placental growth hormone, contribute to the increased insulin resistance in pregnancy.[10] One study found that any impairment of insulin sensitivity existing before pregnancy, in addition to physiologic adaptations to pregnancy, causes significant stress on pancreatic β cells, which leads to more severe deterioration of metabolic state.[8] Even women who develop GDM later in pregnancy have been shown to have deteriorated β cell function in early pregnancy suggesting that a compensatory mechanism for insulin resistance becomes defective early in pregnancy.[8]

Obesity, one of the predominant risk factors for development of GDM, has been studied and characterized as a chronic state of inflammation. Pregnancy, obesity, and GDM are all associated with increased inflammatory markers.[5,11] The placenta is a source of inflammation; in obesity, the placenta is a source of inflammatory cytokines.[5] Current literature and studies support use of inflammatory and other biomarkers to advance understanding of the pathophysiology surrounding GDM.[11] TNF-α and interleukin-6 (IL-6) are manufactured by adipose tissue monocytes and macrophages leading to insulin resistance.[11] Placental production of these proinflammatory cytokines contributes to pregnancy-related insulin resistance.[5,11]

Adipokines exhibit insulin-sensitizing and anti-inflammatory properties. These proteins, secreted from adipocytes, are believed to have prognostic and pathophysiologic significance in GDM due to their metabolic influence on glucose regulation and lipid metabolism.[12,13] Several other hormones including leptin, adiponectin, adipocyte fatty acid-binding protein (AFABP), retinol-binding protein-4, resistin, and visfatin may all play a role in the development and risk for GDM.[11] Leptin is a hormone that increases insulin sensitivity by influencing insulin secretion, glucose utilization, glycogen synthesis, and fatty acid metabolism.[12] Leptin is increased 2- to 3-fold in pregnancy, peaking at around 28 weeks gestation.[12] Leptin production is increased even further in pregnant women with GDM.[12] Using a feedback loop, leptin increases production of TNF-α and IL-6, further increasing insulin resistance.[12] Adiponectin has an inverse relationship to insulin resistance and adiponectin increases fatty acid oxidation and inhibits hepatic glucose production.[5,12] Low levels of adiponectin in the third trimester are associated with the presence of GDM independent of maternal weight.[5] Present studies support adiponectin as an independent risk factor of GDM.[5] Obese individuals, those with insulin resistance and/or T2DM have been found to have decreased adiponectin levels.[12] Adiponectin, with increased levels of TNF-α and leptin, are thought to provide a predictive model for development of GDM as adiponectin levels are reduced by proinflammatory cytokines.[5,12] Evidence suggests that IL-6, AFABP, and visfatin may also be predictive of GDM; however, more studies are required.

GDM risk classification based solely on maternal history and clinical risk factors may not identify all high-risk pregnancies and runs the risk of missing GDM cases.[7,11] Selective screening includes risk factors:

- Previous GDM
- Previous large for gestational age baby
- Any type of diabetes mellitus in a first-degree relative
- Prepregnancy adiposities
- High-risk ethnic group (African American, Asian American, Hispanic, Native American, Pacific Islanders)[3,5,7]
- Glucosuria
- Advanced maternal age[7]

Universal screening is becoming more widely recommended and supported. There is emerging evidence for the use of inflammatory and other biomarkers as useful early prediction models for GDM.[5,11]

There is also supporting evidence of an association between vitamin D deficiency/insufficiency and GDM, maternal obesity, and adverse maternal and pregnancy outcomes.[7] Vitamin D receptor (VDR) is present in islet β cells.[14] Vitamin D is thought to act directly on VDR of pancreatic β cells, regulating intracellular calcium, increasing insulin secretion, and attenuating systemic inflammation associated with insulin resistance.[7,14] Some evidence has actually supported the use of high-dose vitamin D in GDM women to reduce insulin resistance.[14] It is unknown if supplementation of vitamin D could help reduce the risk of GDM or improve glycemic control during pregnancy.

DIAGNOSIS

Screening for GDM has been controversial. GDM can occur in women with no risk factors; however, development is much more prevalent in women who are already at increased risk of T2DM or those with metabolic syndrome.

Risk factors include:

- Overweight or obese women (body mass index [BMI] >25)
- Sedentary women
- Previous pregnancy associated with GDM
- History of macrosomia
- History of hypertension
- Maternal age greater than 35 years
- Women with heart disease
- Women with polycystic ovarian syndrome (PCOS)[3,5]

Obesity is linked to an approximate 3-fold increased risk of development of GDM.[11] Highest prevalence of GDM is found in women from South Asia and South East Asia.[15] Ethnicity is considered the biggest nonmodifiable risk factor for GDM.[15]

There is no universal screening guideline when it comes to diagnosis of GDM. Consensus between the American Diabetes Association (ADA), American College of Obstetricians and Gynecologists (ACOG), and the Endocrine Society agree that women who are at high risk of pre-existing diabetes should be screened at their first prenatal visit using criteria for diagnosis of diabetes in nonpregnant adults.[3,6] Those women include overweight and obese women with at least one other additional risk factor (sedentary lifestyle, family history of diabetes, high-risk ethnicity, history of GDM, hypertension, and/or hyperlipidemia).[3] For all other pregnant women, screening for GDM should occur between 24 and 28 weeks gestation. Performing an oral glucose tolerance test (OGTT) earlier in pregnancy is not well tolerated due to the fasting state, multiple lab draws, and complications of nausea and vomiting in early pregnancy.[5] Despite early diagnosis and adequate management, diagnosis of GDM early in pregnancy remains associated with higher risk of adverse pregnancy events when compared with women diagnosed with GDM after 24 weeks gestation.[6] True prevalence of early GDM diagnosis remains unclear due to varying diagnostic and screening criteria.[6] Revised screening criteria endorsed by the International Association of Diabetes and Pregnancy Study Groups (IADPSG) has further exacerbated the growing problem and prevalence of GDM because of lower diagnostic criteria requiring 1 glucose value above the cutoff value instead of 2 above the cutoff during OGTT.[5,10]

The high physiologic turnover of erythrocytes during pregnancy renders the A1c level inadequate as a diagnostic and management tool in GDM.[5,7] O'Conner and colleagues[5] suggested a trimester-specific reference range for A1c due to vulnerability during this time (**Table 1**).

Table 1	
Proposed trimester-specific A1c reference intervals	
Trimester	**Hba1c Reference Interval**
First	4.8%–5.5% (29–37 mmol/mol)
Second	4.4%–5.4% (25–36 mmol/mol)
Third	4.4%–5.4% (25–36 mmol/mol)

Data from Rodrigo N, Glastras S. The Emerging Role of Biomarkers in the Diagnosis of Gestational Diabetes Mellitus. *Journal of Clinical Medicine.* 2018;7(6):120. https://doi.org/10.3390/jcm7060120.

Diagnosis of GDM is made using an OGTT in either a 1-step or 2-step approach. Both the 1-step and 2-step approaches involve obtaining a fasting plasma glucose, administration of glucose, and additional plasma glucose assessments. Diagnostic criteria vary between the 1-step and 2-step approaches.

The 1-step approach administers a dose of 75-g oral glucose. Additional plasma glucose assessments are taken at 1- and 2-hour intervals after administration. Diagnostic criteria are achieved if one or more of the following values are met (**Table 2**):

The 2-step approach involves an initial screening with a 50-g oral glucose challenge, and an additional 3-hour 100-g OGTT if the first step is positive with a glucose level ≥140 mg/dL. The second step includes plasma assessment at 1, 2, and 3 hours after administration of glucose. Diagnosis of GDM is confirmed if 2 or more of the plasma glucose values meet or exceed in either **Table 3** or **Table 4**:

In 2013, the National Institute of Health (NIH) consensus group supported the 2-step approach for diagnosing GDM. There is lack of substantial clinical trials comparing or supporting the 1-step versus the 2-step approach. ACOG guidelines favor use of the 2-step approach following NIH endorsement.[10,16] IADPSG guidelines recommend universal screening in women at 24 to 28 weeks gestation using a 2-h, 75-g OGTT 1-step approach.[10]

Lack of validity in both early pregnancy OGTT and A1c remains a burden in regard to diagnosis of GDM. Biological markers are being investigated as predictive tools to identify GDM and may help in earlier diagnosis and thus better management throughout pregnancy with fewer complications.[5] Clinical biomarkers, which can be obtained early in pregnancy are believed to be useful in complementing existing clinical risk factors identifying women at high risk of GDM.[5] Cost-effectiveness and universal access to biomarker labs may be prohibitive to their use.

TREATMENT

Lifestyle modification and self-monitoring blood glucose (SMBG) are the gold standards and first-line treatment in GDM.[3,7] Lifestyle modifications involve medical nutrition therapy, physical activity, and weight management based on pregestational

Table 2	
One-step approach—75-g oral glucose tolerance test	
Time	**Plasma Glucose**
Fasting	92
1 h	180
2 h	153

Data from Whalen KL, Taylor JR. Gestational Diabetes Mellitus. In: Murphy JE, Lee, M, editors. Pharmacotherapy self-assessment program: Book 1, Endocrine/Nephrology. ACCP; 2017. p. 7-23.

Table 3 Two-step approach, Time-Carpenter-Coustan thresholds	
Time (h)	**Plasma Glucose**
Fasting	95
1	180
2	155
3	140

Data from Whalen KL, Taylor JR. Gestational Diabetes Mellitus. In: Murphy JE, Lee, M, editors. Pharmacotherapy self-assessment program: Book 1, Endocrine/Nephrology. ACCP; 2017. p. 7-23.

weight. Studies suggest that approximately 75% to 80% of women with GDM can achieve adequate control with lifestyle modifications alone.[3] Management of GDM requires a multidisciplinary team-based approach including obstetric and endocrine practitioners, nutritionist and diabetes educators.

Dietary modification is one of the primary strategies of managing GDM; however, adherence to dietary modifications can be challenging despite motivation to change. Adaptation to a new diet late in pregnancy may be difficult for patients to follow, and some dietary restrictions may infringe on cultural roles and beliefs.[17] Therefore, all women diagnosed with GDM should receive nutritional advice from a registered dietician familiar with management of GDM.[2,18] Nutrition therapy should focus on appropriate weight gain and recommendations for achieving normoglycemia without using stringent calorie-restricted diets.[2] The goal is to support maternal, placental, and fetal metabolic needs.[18] It is important that medical nutrition therapy be culturally sensitive and appropriate.[15]

There are no specific guidelines on nutrition therapy in GDM; however, ACOG and the Endocrine Society continue to refer to carbohydrate restriction, 33% to 40% of total calories, as dietary management.[17,18] No guideline has been found superior in regard to maternal and fetal outcomes.[18] More recent evidence has found that carbohydrate restriction may actually lead to increased dietary fat intake and unbalanced macronutrient intake, which supports evidence of a relationship between maternal lipids (triglycerides and free fatty acids) and excess fetal growth.[17] Diets with high fat intake may promote insulin resistance through a pathway related to increased TNF-α and free fatty acids.[17] In humans, maternal triglyceride and free fatty acid levels may be stronger predictors of excess fetal fat accretion than maternal glucose, thus raising a question of whether glycemic management should be the only focus for GDM therapy.[17]

Complex carbohydrates are less likely to cause postprandial hyperglycemia. They also reduce the need for insulin therapy, lower-fasting low-density lipoprotein

Table 4 Two-step approach, Time National Diabetes data group thresholds	
Time (h)	**Plasma Glucose**
Fasting	105
1	190
2	165
3	145

Data from Whalen KL, Taylor JR. Gestational Diabetes Mellitus. In: Murphy JE, Lee, M, editors. Pharmacotherapy self-assessment program: Book 1, Endocrine/Nephrology. ACCP; 2017. p. 7-23.

cholesterol and free fatty acids while improving insulin sensitivity.[17] A randomized controlled trial recently found that the Choosing Health Options in Carbohydrate Energy diet, when compared with a low carbohydrate diet, effectively controlled glucose levels within current treatment targets.[15,17] Some evidence has also supported the use of the Dietary Approaches to Stop Hypertension diet as beneficial in women with GDM as it is similar to a low glycemic index diet.[3] A limitation to all nutritional studies is that diets cannot be blinded to participants introducing a significant source of bias.[18]

Lifestyle modification should focus on physical activity as a key component in GDM management. Physical activity has been proven to be both safe and effective under proper supervision.[19] Physical activity is known to improve insulin sensitivity and reduce both fasting and postprandial glucose concentrations. The ADA, ACOG, and Endocrine Society all support moderate exercise of 30 to 60 minutes duration most days of the week for women with GDM and no medical or obstetric contraindications to physical activity. However, there are no specific guidelines for type of exercise, frequency, intensity, time, or duration for women with GDM.[3,19,20] It is a recommended that an exercise physiologist be consulted for women who have been sedentary before pregnancy.[19] As with any relative contraindication to exercise, advice from the medical provider and an exercise physiologist should be taken into account to weigh risk versus benefits of exercise.[19] Any medical condition that may be exacerbated by exercise is contraindicated.[19] Both aerobic exercise and resistance strength training are safe and effective and lower glucose levels in women with GDM.[19]

Pharmacologic therapy should be initiated if medical nutrition therapy and physical activity guidelines fail to achieve glucose goals in 1 to 2 weeks.[3] Daily SMBG should be performed fasting, 1 hour postprandial, and 2 hour postprandial.[20] **Table 5** outlines recommended glycemic targets in patients with GDM.

Insulin is considered effective and safe for the fetus as insulin does not cross the placenta and, thus, is first-line therapy in GDM.[3] It does, however, increase the risk of hypoglycemia and weight gain.[3] Barriers to insulin therapy can include cost, administration, and patient education. No evidence exists to support any specific insulin regimen as superior during pregnancy; therapy may include multiple daily injections or continuous infusion. Pathophysiology of pregnancy requires frequent titration of insulin with continued daily and frequent SMBG.[3] Insulin therapy can be initiated in several ways including a weight-based dosing, trimester + weight-based dosing, or a standard starting dose for all patients determined by clinician judgment (**Table 6**).[9,10,20]

There are no specific guidelines for the initiation of insulin therapy, the dose, the frequency, or the titration.[9] Insulin analogs have a more physiologic profile than human insulins.

Table 5 Recommended glycemic targets for patients with gestational diabetes			
Guideline	Fasting	1 h Postprandial	2 h Postprandial
ACOG	≤95	<140	<120
ADA	≤95	≤140	≤120
Endocrine Society	≤95	≤140	≤120
NICE (National Institute for Health & Care Excellence)	≤95	<140	<115

Data from Whalen KL, Taylor JR. Gestational Diabetes Mellitus. In: Murphy JE, Lee, M, editors. Pharmacotherapy self-assessment program: Book 1, Endocrine/Nephrology. ACCP; 2017. p. 7-23.

Table 6	
Trimester + weight-based dosing for initiation of insulin therapy	
Trimester	Total Daily Dose (units/kg)
First	0.7
Second	0.8
Third	0.9–1

Data from Blum AK. Insulin Use in Pregnancy: An Update. *Diabetes Spectrum*. 2016;29(2):92-97. https://doi.org/10.2337/diaspect.29.2.92.

These insulins carry a US Food and Drug Administration (FDA) category B rating, meaning that the FDA has received sufficient human data to deem them low risk in pregnancy.[9]

- Regular insulin (U-100 and U-500 concentrations)
- Insulin aspart
- Insulin lispro
- Neutral protamine Hagedorn
- Insulin detemir

Insulin glulisine, insulin degludec, and inhaled human insulin carry a category C rating, meaning there are no human data during pregnancy.[9] Insulin glargine has been a somewhat controversial topic regarding use in pregnancy; however, there is no conclusive evidence for any increased adverse reactions associated with its use in pregnancy.[10] For those insulin analogs that lack any sufficient human data, one must take into account risk assessment when deciding on an insulin regimen.[9]

A large randomized controlled trial performed by Rowan and colleagues[7,10,21] concluded that metformin, alone or with supplemental insulin, was not associated with increased perinatal complications compared with insulin alone; therefore, treatment with metformin was considered safe and effective. Metformin has been found to have a lower risk of neonatal hypoglycemia and less maternal weight gain than insulin in systemic reviews.[3] However, metformin does cross the placenta. Metformin is also associated with slightly increased risk of prematurity and higher BMI and obesity in the baby.[3,20] Use of metformin should be reserved for those women who are unable to take insulin therapy or who decline/refuse use of insulin therapy.[22] There are no long-term studies in the use of metformin in GDM and women should be counseled appropriately.[7] Before starting metformin treatment, baseline kidney function should be checked and women should be counseled regarding the side effects.

Often the patient with PCOS is prescribed metformin before conception. There is no benefit to continue metformin during pregnancy for these women as there is no evidence that metformin will present spontaneous abortion or GDM.[3] In addition, there is no reported adverse effects to the fetus in PCOS women who have been treated with metformin for infertility.[10]

A randomized control trial compared use of glyburide versus insulin and found no significant differences between the glyburide and insulin groups regarding macrosomia, neonatal hypoglycemia, lung complications, or fetal abnormalities.[7] This study concluded that glyburide is a clinically effective alternative to insulin therapy.[7] However, the ADA 2019 Standards of Care Guidelines stated glyburide was associated with an increased risk of neonatal hypoglycemia and macrosomia compared with use of metformin or insulin.[3,23] Use of glyburide should be avoided in place of insulin.[22,23] Glyburide is known to cross the placenta (concentrations in umbilical cord plasma are approximately 70% of maternal levels).[3] With glyburide, long-term safety data for the baby is not available.

A study of the efficacy and safety of glyburide and metformin in GDM found both treatments to be comparable.[21] This trial looked at the usefulness and potential for treatment with the addition of a second oral hypoglycemic agent (OHA) as second-line therapy during treatment failure, with insulin only reserved for third-line therapy.[21] It was hypothesized during this trial that, due to the different mechanisms of action between metformin and glyburide, the addition of the second OHA would compensate when the first agent had failed.[21] This strategy was found to increase treatment success from 69% to 89%, with only 11% of the patient requiring insulin therapy.[21] This study concluded that the combination of metformin and glyburide allows for a higher efficacy rate and a reduced need for insulin. Insulin was reserved for patients who have failed to respond to both medications or who experienced adverse events.[21] However, not only are there possible adverse reactions to glyburide and metformin, but there is a paucity of long-term follow-up data on both mother and offspring regarding these therapies.[7]

INTRAPARTUM CARE

There are no clear or universal guidelines for timing of delivery in GDM pregnancies. A handful of studies support inducing insulin-treated women at 38 to 39 weeks.[10] Other literature supports induction of labor before 39 weeks but only if glycemic control is poor or another indication for induction is present.[20] Women with ultrasound screenings showing macrosomia should also undergo induction at 38 to 39 weeks.[10] For women with GDM who have an estimated fetal weight greater than 4500 g (9 lbs, 14 oz), scheduled cesarean delivery should be considered to reduce the risk of permanent birth injury.[20] There are no indications to pursue delivery earlier than 40 weeks in patients with well controlled glycemic levels.

During labor and delivery, maintain normal glucose level between 72 and 126 mg/dL to prevent neonatal hypoglycemia.[10] Patients should continue to undergo frequent glucose monitoring; those not on insulin should be monitored every 4 to 6 hours, and women treated with insulin therapy should be monitored every 2 hours.[10,20] Dextrose fluids should be used to treat women with hypoglycemia. Insulin infusion should be initiated to maintain target glycemic levels in women with glucose exceeding 140 mg/dL.[10]

POSTPARTUM CARE

Fasting blood glucose should be monitored for 24 to 72 hours after delivery to assure hyperglycemia has resolved.[10] Most women with GDM will be able to resume their prepregnancy diet, and 95% of women with GDM will return to euglycemia after delivery without need for further treatment.[10,20] Those women found to have overt diabetes after delivery should be managed accordingly. Guidelines have shown that women with overt diabetes who have used metformin or glyburide therapy with pregnancy can continue this regimen during breastfeeding, if necessary.[10]

GDM is associated with an increased maternal lifetime risk for T2DM, estimated as 50% to 75% of women after 15 to 25 years.[3] These women are also at higher risk for metabolic syndrome and CVD. Women with GDM should be tested for persistent diabetes or prediabetes at 6 to 12 weeks postpartum using a 75-g OGTT and nonpregnancy criteria.[3] OGTT is recommended over A1c at 6 to 12 weeks postpartum as A1c levels may be persistently affected by increased red blood cell turnover, therefore making the OGTT a more sensitive test.[3,10] Continued testing is recommended every

1 to 3 years if the OGTT is normal and can be followed with an A1c level.[3] Intensive lifestyle management and/or treatment with metformin may prevent and/or delay progression to T2DM.

SUMMARY

The prevalence of GDM continues to increase worldwide due to increasing obesity rates, prevalence of insulin resistance and T2DM, advancing maternal age, and changes in screening criteria. GDM has been shown to have both short-term and long-term adverse actions on both the mother and fetus and is highly associated with poorer pregnancy outcomes. The pathophysiology behind GDM remains unknown, but seems based in increased BMI, insulin resistance, and inflammatory pathways. Because of the effects on the pregnancy, the mother, and offspring long term, there has been a call for universal screening for GDM. Newer guidelines suggest screening of high-risk women early in pregnancy. There are limitations in early diagnosis and recognition of GDM, thus opening the door to use of biomarkers in the future to help better identify and manage patients with GDM. Despite advancements, additional GDM research needs to define a better understanding of pathophysiology, screening, diagnosis, and best approaches to treatment.

DISCLOSURE

The author has nothing to disclosure.

REFERENCES

1. HAPO Study Cooperative Research Group, Metzger BE, Lowe LP, Dyer AR, et al. Hyperglycemia and adverse pregnancy outcomes. N Engl J Med 2008;358(19): 1991–2002.
2. Kaaja R, Rönnemaa T. Gestational diabetes: pathogenesis and consequences to mother and offspring. Rev Diabet Stud 2008;5(4):194–202.
3. American Diabetes Association. Management of diabetes in pregnancy: standards of medical care in diabetes – 2019. Diabetes Care 2019;42(Suppl 1): S165–72.
4. Centers for Disease Control and Prevention. Gestational diabetes and pregnancy | CDC. Atlanta (GA): US Department of Health and Human Services. Available at: https://www.cdc.gov/pregnancy/diabetes-gestational.html. Accessed March 3, 2019.
5. Rodrigo N, Glastras S. The emerging role of biomarkers in the diagnosis of gestational diabetes mellitus. J Clin Med 2018;7(6) [pii:E120].
6. Sweeting AN, Ross GP, Hyett J, et al. Gestational diabetes mellitus in early pregnancy: evidence for poor pregnancy outcomes despite treatment. Diabetes Care 2016;39(1):75–81.
7. Kampmann U, Madsen LR, Skajaa GO, et al. Gestational diabetes: a clinical update. World J Diabetes 2015;6(8):1065–72.
8. Bozkurt L, Göbl CS, Pfligl L, et al. Pathophysiological characteristics and effects of obesity in women with early and late manifestation of gestational diabetes diagnosed by the International Association of Diabetes and Pregnancy Study Groups criteria. J Clin Endocrinol Metab 2015;100(3):1113–20.
9. Blum AK. Insulin use in pregnancy: an update. Diabetes Spectr 2016;29(2):92–7.
10. Alfadhli E. Gestational diabetes mellitus. Saudi Med J 2015;36(4):399–406.

11. Abell S, De Courten BD, Boyle J, et al. Inflammatory and other biomarkers: role in pathophysiology and prediction of gestational diabetes mellitus. Int J Mol Sci 2015;16(6):13442–73.
12. Al-Badri MR, Zantout MS, Azar ST. The role of adipokines in gestational diabetes mellitus. Ther Adv Endocrinol Metab 2015;6(3):103–8.
13. Tsiotra PC, Halvatsiotis P, Patsouras K, et al. Circulating adipokines and mRNA expression in adipose tissue and the placenta in women with gestational diabetes mellitus. Peptides 2018;101:157–66.
14. Zhang Q, Cheng Y, He M, et al. Effect of various doses of vitamin D supplementation on pregnant women with gestational diabetes mellitus: a randomized controlled trial. Exp Ther Med 2016;12(3):1889–95.
15. Yuen L, Wong VW. Gestational diabetes mellitus: challenges for different ethnic groups. World J Diabetes 2015;6(8):1024–32.
16. Committee on Practice Bulletins—Obstetrics. ACOG practice bulletin no. 190: gestational diabetes mellitus. Obstet Gynecol 2018;131(2):e49–64.
17. Hernandez TL. Carbohydrate content in the GDM diet: two views: view 1: nutrition therapy in gestational diabetes: the case for complex carbohydrates. Diabetes Spectr 2016;29(2):82–8.
18. Hernandez TL, Brand-Miller JC. Nutrition therapy in gestational diabetes mellitus: time to move forward. Diabetes Care 2018;41(7):1343–5.
19. Padayachee C, Coombes JS. Exercise guidelines for gestational diabetes mellitus. World J Diabetes 2015;6(8):1033–44.
20. Garrison A. Screening, diagnosis, and management of gestational diabetes mellitus. Am Fam Physician 2015;91(7):460–7.
21. Nachum Z, Zafran N, Salim R, et al. Glyburide versus metformin and their combination for the treatment of gestational diabetes mellitus: a randomized controlled study. Diabetes Care 2017;40(3):332–7.
22. Whalen KL, Taylor JR. Gestational diabetes mellitus. In: Murphy JE, Lee M, editors. Pharmacotherapy self-assessment program: book 1, endocrine/nephrology. Lenexa: ACCP; 2017. p. 7–23.
23. Camelo Castillo W, Boggess K, Stürmer T, et al. Association of adverse pregnancy outcomes with glyburide vs insulin in women with gestational diabetes. JAMA Pediatr 2015;169(5):452–8.

Sugar Babies
Diabetes in the Pediatric Population

Molly E. Band, MHS, PA-C

KEYWORDS

- Type 1 diabetes • Pediatric • Adolescent • Transition to adult care

KEY POINTS

- Type 1 diabetes mellitus is the most common form of diabetes in the pediatric population.
- The incidence of type 1 and 2 diabetes mellitus is increasing in the pediatric population.
- The management of diabetes in children should be team based and developmentally appropriate based on the child's age.

INTRODUCTION

Diabetes mellitus (DM) is a complex group of metabolic disorders characterized by a chronically elevated blood glucose level, which can result from either a defect in insulin secretion, a defect in insulin responsiveness, or both.[1,2] Although there are many similarities between diabetes in adults and diabetes in children, there are significant differences in diagnosis, presentation, and treatment in the pediatric population. This article focuses on pediatric-specific aspects of diabetes.

DEFINITION AND DIAGNOSIS

The diagnostic criteria of DM (**Box 1**) in children is based on blood glucose measurements in the presence or absence of symptoms (**Table 1**). A challenging piece to the diagnosis of DM is that, based on age and development, the signs and symptoms in young infants and children may be difficult to detect. Thus, the diagnosis of DM can be overlooked, delayed, or mistaken for something else. Examples include diagnosing a child with pneumonia or asthma if there is labored breathing; diagnosing a child with appendicitis or gastroenteritis if there is abdominal pain and vomiting; diagnosing a child with a urinary tract infection if there is urinary frequency and enuresis, and so forth.[2,3]

Department of Pediatric Nephrology, Connecticut Children's Medical Center, 282 Washington Street, Suite 2J, Hartford, CT 06106, USA
E-mail address: mband@connecticutchildrens.org

Physician Assist Clin 5 (2020) 237–246
https://doi.org/10.1016/j.cpha.2019.11.007
physicianassistant.theclinics.com

<table>
<tr><td>

Box 1
American Diabetes Association diagnostic criteria

Symptoms of diabetes with plasma glucose concentration $\geq$11.1 mmol/L (200 mg/dL)

OR

Fasting (no caloric intake for 8 hours) plasma glucose greater than 7.0 mmol/L (126 mg/dL)

OR

Two-hour postload glucose greater than 11.1 mmol/L (200 mg/dL) on an oral glucose tolerance test (1.75 g/kg of body weight to a maximum of 75-g glucose load)

OR

Hemoglobin A1c greater than 6.5%

Data from Refs.[1,2,4]
</td></tr>
</table>

CLASSIFICATION OF DIABETES IN THE PEDIATRIC POPULATION

The clinical presentation guides the assignment of children into types of diabetes, which has become increasingly challenging given the rising prevalence of overweight and obesity in the pediatric population.[1] Most children with DM will have type 1 diabetes mellitus (T1DM), which accounts for more than 90% of childhood and adolescent diabetes in most western countries, although the incidence of type 2 diabetes mellitus (T2DM) is increasing. In contrast, T1DM accounts for 5% to 10% of diabetes across the adult lifespan.[1]

Type 1 Diabetes Mellitus

T1DM is characterized by chronic immune-mediated destruction of pancreatic β-cells and is the most common autoimmune disorder in the youth.[1,2] The destruction of β-cells occurs at variable rates and leads to insulin deficiency.

The cause of T1DM is multifactorial with genetic predisposition and environmental factors playing a role, although the mechanism is not fully understood.[1,2] Diabetes-associated autoantibodies include GAD, IA2, IAA, and ZnT8. Susceptibility to T1DM is determined by multiple genes with HLA genotype conferring about 30% to 50% of risk.[1,3] Having a first-degree relative with T1DM leads to an approximately 15-fold increased relative lifetime risk of developing T1DM, although conversely, 85%

Table 1 **Signs and symptoms**	
Diabetes Mellitus	**Diabetic Ketoacidosis**
Weight loss	Abdominal pain/vomiting
Polydipsia (excessive thirst)	Fruity smell on breath
Polyphagia (excessive hunger)	Severe dehydration
Polyuria, enuresis	Altered mental status
Fatigue	Kussmaul breathing (deep, rapid, sighing)
Altered mood	Shock
Thrush	Coma

Data from Pocketbook for management of diabetes in childhood and adolescence in under-resourced countries, 2nd edition, International Diabetes Federation, Brussels, 2017.

of children do not have a family history of T1DM. Environmental factors are largely unknown, but can include dietary, infectious, or psychosocial factors. Examples include congenital rubella syndrome and other viruses, including enterovirus, cytomegalovirus, mumps, influenza, and rotavirus.[1,5]

Overall, it is estimated that 96,000 children under the age of 15 years will develop T1DM annually worldwide, and there are currently 500,000 children living with T1DM worldwide. The incidence of T1DM varies across demographic subgroups, including age, sex, and race or ethnic groups, with the highest incidence rates in Finland, Northern Europe, and Canada, with very low incidence rates in Asia. T1DM is found more frequently in male children than in female children.[1] A study by Mayer-Davis and colleagues[5] revealed that from 2002 to 2012 there was a significant upward trend in the incidence of T1DM with an annual increase of 1.4%. This increase is likely due to factors not yet identified but speculated to be both environmental and behavioral factors.

There are distinct, identifiable stages that the youth progress through before becoming symptomatic (**Tables 2** and **3**).[1,3]

Type 2 Diabetes Mellitus

T2DM has characteristics and features that are distinct and unique to the pediatric population. The cause of T2DM differs from that of T1DM in that there is not an identified autoimmune process; rather, insulin secretion is not sufficient to meet the demand.

T2DM is diagnosed in the youth population using standard American Diabetes Association (ADA) criteria (see **Box 1**), but pediatric patients also need determination of diabetes type. All pediatric patients presenting with new-onset diabetes should have diabetes autoantibody testing, because positive testing can predict the rate of development of insulin requirements. Additional evaluation should include screening for hypertension, dyslipidemia, elevated liver enzymes, and microalbuminuria. Patients should also be screened for obstructive sleep apnea and mental health disorders, including anxiety, depression, and eating disorders.[6]

Epidemiologic data in children and adolescents are less robust than in the adult population, but the incidence of T2DM varies among geographic location, age, and ethnicity. The incidence ranges from 1 to 51 per 1000, with the highest in North American Indians aged 15 to 19 years.[1] Similar to that of T1DM, the incidence has significantly increased at a relative annual increase of 4.8% from the time period of 2002 to 2012, as shown by Mayer-Davis and colleagues.[5] This increase was noted in all racial and ethnic groups except non-Hispanic whites. Risk factors for developing T2DM in the pediatric population include obesity, family history of T2DM, and being of certain ethnic and genetic backgrounds.[1] The median age of youth-onset T2DM is 13.5 years and rarely occurs before puberty.[6]

Table 2	
Stages of type 1 diabetes mellitus	
Stage	**Characteristic**
1	Multiple islet antibodies, normal blood glucose, presymptomatic
2	Multiple islet antibodies, raised blood glucose, and presymptomatic
3	Islet autoimmunity, raised blood glucose, and symptomatic
4	Long-standing T1DM

Data from Refs.[1,3]

Table 3	
When to consider monogenic diabetes mellitus	
Consider in the Following Scenarios for Patients Diagnosed with T2DM	**Consider in the Following Scenarios for Patients Diagnosed with T2DM**
• DM presenting under 6 mo of age • DM presenting between ages 6 and 12 mo without evidence of autoimmunity or if other congenital defects or unusual family history of present	• Lack of severe obesity
• Family history of DM in 1 parent and first degree relative of affected parent	• Family history of DM in 1 parent and first degree relative of affected parent
• Lack of islet autoantibodies	• Lack of acanthosis nigricans and/or other features of metabolic syndrome
• Preserved β-cell function • Low insulin requirements • Detectable C-peptide	• Unusual fat distribution

Data from Hattersley AT, Greeley SA, Plak M, et al. ISPAD clinical practice consensus guidelines 2018: the diagnosis and management of monogenic diabetes in children and adolescents. *Pediatr Diabetes* 2018:19 Suppl 27: 47-63.

Monogenic Diabetes Mellitus

Monogenic DM occurs when there is one or more defects in a single gene and can be inherited as a dominant or recessive, non-Mendelian trait, or as a spontaneous mutation. Although monogenic DM is rare, accounting for 1% to 6% of pediatric diabetes patients, it holds important treatment and prognostic implications if identified. There are currently more than 40 subtypes of monogenic DM, with the 2 main categories being neonatal DM and maturity-onset DM.[7,8]

Cystic Fibrosis-Related Diabetes

Cystic fibrosis (CF) -related diabetes (CFRD) occurs secondary to insulin and glucagon deficiency, as well as insulin resistance, which can be related to acute illnesses and medications. It is the most common comorbidity associated with CF. CFRD can occur at any age, but most commonly occurs in adolescence and early adulthood. Because of the increased morbidity and mortality, annual screening for CFRD should start by age 10 in all CF patients.[1]

TREATMENT
Diabetic Education

The proposed definition of diabetes education is *Diabetes education is an interactive process that facilitates and supports the individual and/or their families, those who provide care or significant social contacts to acquire and apply the knowledge, confidence, and practical, problem solving and coping skills, needed to manage their life with diabetes in order to achieve the best possible outcomes within their own unique circumstances.*[9]

Diabetes education should be provided to patients and their caregivers by a multidisciplinary team at diagnosis and throughout the course of treatment. It should be adapted based on the patient's age and developmental stage, stage of diabetes, culture, and learning pace. It should be provided in the family's native language. Education, especially for the pediatric population, is a critical element of diabetes treatment and has been proven to be cost-effective by reducing the frequency of emergency department visits and hospitalizations.[9]

Nutritional Management

Nutritional management is an essential component in the treatment of all patients with diabetes, even more so in the pediatric population. Nutritional education is ideally provided by a specialist pediatric dietitian with experience in childhood diabetes. It should be individualized based on the child and family's culture and psychosocial needs, which may change throughout the course of childhood. The dietitian should develop a trusting and supportive relationship with the child and family for optimal results.

The aims of nutritional management should include the following:

- Healthy eating habits that can be maintained among the family for life should be encouraged
- Three meals a day from all food groups and healthy snacks when appropriate with discouragement from binge-eating
- Sufficient nutrients for optimal growth, development, and good health
- Balance between intake and metabolic requirements[10]

Insulin

Children and adolescents with T1DM are dependent on insulin therapy for treatment. Insulin should be started ideally within 6 hours after diagnosis particularly if Ketonuria is present. The purpose of insulin therapy is to improve glycemic control and minimize the risks of acute and chronic complications of diabetes. Over the last several decades, there has been a change in the recommendation regarding the frequency of insulin dosing in children. Previously, the goal was to minimize painful injections; however, more recent studies support more frequent injections and an intensive insulin regimen. The absorption of insulin varies in children and adolescents compared with adults. A key point is that younger children typically have less subcutaneous fat and therefore faster absorption and shorter duration of action.[11]

COMPLICATIONS

There are some differences in the complications of DM in the pediatric population when comparing outcomes of T1DM versus T2DM. The focus here is primarily on complications of T1DM, although T2DM will be included in the discussion.

Diabetic Ketoacidosis

There are several studies whereby diabetic ketoacidosis (DKA) has occurred in patients with T2DM at diagnosis. There are also reports of hyperglycemic hyperosmolar state in children with T2DM.[12] DKA at disease onset occurs in approximately 15% to 70% of children with T1DM in Europe and North America. It is more common in younger children, in ethnic minority groups, and in children with limited access to medical care. The risk of DKA in children with established T1DM is 1% to 10% per year. Risk factors include omission of insulin, poor diabetic control, prior episodes of DKA, psychiatric disorders, including eating disorders, unstable family circumstances, pubertal and adolescent girls, binge alcohol ingestion, and limited access to medical care.[13]

Hypoglycemia

Hypoglycemia is the most common acute complication in children and adolescents with T2DM but can also occur in T2DM. Although a glucose level less than 70 mg/dL is an alert value for hypoglycemia, there is not a single glucose value to define hypoglycemia. Hypoglycemic symptoms can occur when plasma glucose concentrations shift to lower than that of the individual's glycemic thresholds. **Table 4** describes the varying degrees of hypoglycemia. Causes of hypoglycemia include excessive insulin dosing, decreased food consumption, exercise, sleep, and alcohol ingestion. The symptoms of hypoglycemia can include shakiness, sweatiness, poor concentration, slurred speech, poor judgment, confusion, irritability, inconsolable crying, and tiredness. Young children are at higher risk for severe hypoglycemia compared with older age groups because of their lower ability to communicate their symptoms.

Microvascular and Macrovascular Complications

Diabetes-related vascular complications include nephropathy, retinopathy, neuropathy, and macrovascular disease (**Table 5**). Although clinically evident complications are less common in children, early changes may be detectable within a few years of diagnosis of DM. The goal of screening for these complications is to prevent or delay the onset and progression. The risk of development of these complications can be reduced with intensive diabetic treatment and improved glycemic control.[14]

Growth and Development

Monitoring growth with anthropometric measurements is an important part of routine care in patients with diabetes because suboptimal glycemic control has been associated with a decrease in height velocity. Girls are at higher risk for being overweight compared with boys, and menarche may be delayed.[15]

Other Autoimmune Disorders

Children with T1DM are at an increased risk for developing other autoimmune disorders compared with their peers. About 25% of pediatric patients with T1DM will also be diagnosed with another autoimmune disorder. Although there is a wide range of comorbid autoimmune disorders, thyroid disease and celiac disease are the most common.[15]

Table 4 Definition of hypoglycemia	
Hypoglycemia	**Clinical Information**
Clinical hypoglycemia alert	• Glucose <70 • There is potential for glucose to drop further and corrective action is needed
Clinically important or serious hypoglycemia	• Glucose <54 • These levels may lead to impaired awareness of hypoglycemia • There is an increased risk of severe hypoglycemia
Severe hypoglycemia	• An event associated with severe cognitive impairment that requires external assistance to administer corrective treatment

Data from Abraham MB, Jones TW, Naranjo D, et al. ISPAD clinical practice consensus guidelines 2018: assessment and management of hypoglycemia in children and adolescents with diabetes. *Pediatr Diabetes* 2018;19 Suppl 27:178-192.

Table 5
Microvascular and macrovascular complications of diabetes mellitus

Organ System	Manifestations	Screening
Diabetic nephropathy	• Kidney failure • Hypertension	• Urinary albumin/creatinine ratio
Diabetic retinopathy	• Visual impairment • Blindness	• Fundal photography or mydriatic ophthalmoscopy
Diabetic autonomic neuropathy	• Postural hypotension • Gastroparesis • Diarrhea • Bladder impairment • Impotence	• History • Physical examination • Clinical tests
Diabetic peripheral neuropathy	• Pain • Paresthesia • Muscle weakness	• History • Physical examination • Clinical tests
Diabetic macrovascular disease	• Cardiac disease • Peripheral vascular disease • Stroke	• Lipid profile every 2 y • BP annually

Abbreviation: BP, blood pressure.
Data from Donaghue KC, Marcovecchio ML, Wadwa RP, et al. ISPAD clinical practice consensus guidelines 2018: microvascular and macrovascular complications in children and adolescents. *Pediatr Diabetes* 2018: 19 Suppl. 27:: 262-274.

- Autoimmune thyroid disease
  - Hashimoto thyroiditis
  - Graves disease
- Celiac disease
- Primary adrenal insufficiency (Addison disease)
- Collagen vascular disease
  - Rheumatoid arthritis
  - Lupus
  - Psoriasis
  - Scleroderma
- Autoimmune gastric disease
  - Crohn disease
  - Ulcerative colitis
  - Autoimmune hepatitis
  - Autoimmune gastritis
- Autoimmune skin disease
  - Vitiligo
  - Alopecia
  - Scleroderma

DIABETES IN SCHOOL

Children and adolescents spend a significant amount of their time at school, accounting for up to 8 to 10 hours per day. During this time, the child is under the supervision of school personnel, including teachers, school nurses, and administrators. Thus, it is imperative that school personnel have adequate and appropriate training on how to care for children with diabetes. This training includes routine care (blood glucose monitoring, administration of insulin, nutrition) as well as acute care for consequences of diabetes (hyperglycemia, hypoglycemia).[16]

To provide guidance to school personnel on the care of a child or adolescent with diabetes, each child should have an individualized diabetes management plan (DMP). The DMP is outlined by the parent/child and the diabetes health care team and is provided to the school. This DMP should be updated and reviewed on an annual basis, or sooner if changes are necessary as determined by the health care team. The DMP should include the child's identification information, contact information for the child's parents/guardians as well as health care team, what time the blood glucose should be monitored, target ranges for glucose measurements, type of insulin treatment and device, guidance to dose adjustments, symptoms and treatment for hyperglycemic or hypoglycemic episodes, information on a meal plan, information regarding activities and exercise, and so forth.[16]

Blood glucose monitoring is essential to maintain appropriate levels throughout the course of the day. Several factors can affect blood glucose, including the degree of the child's physical activity and/or stress level. Blood glucose monitoring should be performed before each meal, before and after physical activity, as well as before testing/examinations. Glucose is essential for central nervous system functioning; thus, diabetes and alterations in glucose have the potential to affect a child's cognition. Hypoglycemic effects include hindering problem-solving skills, loss of consciousness, or seizures. Hyperglycemic effects include decreased ability to concentrate and/or decreased cognitive function.[16]

DIABETES IN ADOLESCENCE AND TRANSITION TO ADULT CARE

Adolescence (ages 13–19 years) is a period of transition from childhood to adulthood and oftentimes includes unique developmental challenges. Adolescents with chronic diseases, including both T1DM and T2DM, have an additional challenge in successfully transitioning their diabetes care from a pediatric provider to an adult provider. With the increasing prevalence of diabetes, there currently is, and will continue to be, increasing numbers of young adults who will require transition of care. Although the physical transition from pediatric to adult care often does not happen until after the patient is older than 18 years of age, discussions surrounding transition should occur with both the patient and the family beginning in early adolescence. This discussion will help to prepare all parties on the expectations surrounding independent diabetes care and transition to adult providers.

The term "emerging adults" references the time span from the ages of 18 to 30 years. It is a high-risk time period for patients with DM with an increased risk for poor glycemic control, gaps in medical care, and known complications of diabetes. There are often multiple competing priorities for patients in this age range, including educational, social/emotional, occupational, and financial priorities, all of which can negatively impact diabetes care. Hemoglobin A1c target for patients aged 13 to 18 years is 7.5% and less than 7% for patients older than 19 years. Less than one-third of patients aged 13 to 18 years met this goal, and less than 20% of patients aged greater than 19 years achieved these targets.[17]

Recommendations for adult providers to enable a successful transition from pediatric to adult care include the following[18]:

1. Communicate with pediatric colleagues before, during, and after transition to coordinate care and minimize gaps
2. Assess objectively knowledge and skills levels, which can help the adult provider capitalize on strengths and identify needs for intervention

3. Focus on establishing a relationship, not just perfecting A1c
4. Develop a strategy in your clinic to routinely identify and address psychosocial needs for young adult patients
5. Applying a team-based approach can help young adults stay engaged

SUMMARY

In children, the most common form of DM is T1DM, which results from a destruction of β-cells. T2DM is becoming more prevalent in the pediatric population with an increasing incidence owing to the obesity epidemic. The treatment of DM in children varies based on cause. Management of diabetes in the pediatric patient should be multidisciplinary and include the parents or primary caregivers, medical providers, dietitians, and school personnel. Adolescence and the emerging adult periods can be a challenging transition for many patients with a higher risk for poor diabetic control.

DISCLOSURE

M.E. Band has nothing to disclose.

REFERENCES

1. Mayer-Davis EJ, Kahkoska AR, Jefferies C, et al. ISPAD clinical practice consensus guidelines 2018: definition, epidemiology, and classification of diabetes in children and adolescents. Pediatr Diabetes 2018;19(Suppl 27):7–19.
2. Ogle G, Middlehurst A, Silink M, et al. Pocketbook for management of diabetes in childhood and adolescence in under-resourced countries. 2nd edition. Brussels (Belgium): International Diabetes Federation; 2017.
3. Couper JJ, Haller MJ, Greenbaum CJ, et al. ISPAD clinical practice consensus guidelines 2018: stages of type 1 diabetes in children and adolescents. Pediatr Diabetes 2018;19(Suppl 27):20–7.
4. Chiang JL, Kirkman MS, Laffel LMB, et al. Type 1 diabetes through the life span: a position statement of the American Diabetes Association. Diabetes Care 2014;34: 2034–54.
5. Mayer-Davis EJ, Lawrence JM, Dabelea D, et al. Incidence trends of type 1 and type 2 diabetes among youths, 2002-2012. N Engl J Med 2017;376:1419–29.
6. Zeitler P, Arslanian S, Fr J, et al. ISPAD clinical practice consensus guidelines 2018: type 2 diabetes mellitus in youth. Pediatr Diabetes 2018;19(Suppl 27): 28–46.
7. Hattersley AT, Greeley SA, Plak M, et al. ISPAD clinical practice consensus guidelines 2018: the diagnosis and management of monogenic diabetes in children and adolescents. Pediatr Diabetes 2018;19(Suppl 27):47–63.
8. Steck AK, Winter WE. Review on monogenic diabetes. Curr Opin Endocrinol Diabetes Obes 2011;18:252–8.
9. Phelan H, Lange K, Cengiz E, et al. ISPAD clinical practice consensus guidelines 2018: diabetes education in children and adolescents. Pediatr Diabetes 2018; 19(Suppl 27):75–83.
10. Smart CE, Annan F, Higgins LA, et al. ISPAD Clinical Practice Consensus Guidelines 2018: nutritional management in children and adolescents with diabetes. Pediatr Diabetes 2018;19(Suppl 27):136–54.

11. Danne T, Phillip M, Buckingham BA. ISPAD clinical practice consensus guidelines 2018: insulin treatment in children and adolescents with diabetes. Pediatr Diabetes 2018;19(Suppl 27):115–35.
12. Pinhas-Hamiel O, Zeitler P. Acute and chronic complications of type 2 diabetes mellitus in children and adolescents. Lancet 2007;369:1823–31.
13. Wolfsdorf JI, Glase N, Agus M, et al. ISPAD clinical practice consensus guidelines 2018: diabetic ketoacidosis and the hyperglycemic hyperosmolar state. Pediatr Diabetes 2018;19(Suppl 27):155–77.
14. Donaghue KC, Marcovecchio ML, Wadwa RP, et al. ISPAD clinical practice consensus guidelines 2018: microvascular and macrovascular complications in children and adolescents. Pediatr Diabetes 2018;19(Suppl. 27):262–74.
15. Mahmud FH, Elbarbary NS, Frohlich-Reiterer E, et al. ISPAD clinical practice consensus guidelines 2018: other complications and associated conditions in children and adolescents with type 1 diabetes. Pediatr Diabetes 2018;19(Suppl. 27):275–86.
16. Bratina N, Forsander G, Annan F, et al. ISPAD clinical practice consensus guidelines 2018: management and support of children and adolescents with type 1 diabetes in school. Pediatr Diabetes 2018;19(Suppl 27):287–301.
17. Garvey KC, Markowitz JT, Laffel LMB. Transition to adult care for youth with type 1 diabetes. Curr Diab Rep 2012;12(5):533–41.
18. Iyengar J, Thomas IN, Soleimanpour SA. Transition from pediatric to adult care in emerging adults with type 1 diabetes: a blueprint for effective receivership. Clin Diabetes Endocrinol 2019;5(3):1–7.

The Boomers Come of Age
The Elderly and Frail Patients

Ashley Klaczak Mudra, MPAS, PA-C

KEYWORDS

- Elderly • Diabetes mellitus • T2DM • T1DM • Oral antidiabetic drugs • Insulin
- Hypoglycemia • Nursing homes

KEY POINTS

- Diabetes mellitus, specifically type 2, is becoming more prevalent in the United States, especially in the population over the age of 65 years.
- Functional status, cognitive impairment, screening for depression, risk of hypoglycemia, falling risk, and polypharmacy are factors to consider while managing diabetes in those with advancing age.
- Individualize glycemia targets to optimize blood glucose levels while considering functional status and life expectancy.
- A multidisciplinary team with primary care, endocrinology, and diabetes educators is essential for the education, prevention, recognition, and individualized diabetic treatment plan in the elderly population.

INTRODUCTION

As a health consequence of the worldwide obesity epidemic nearly tripling since 1975 according to the World Health Organization, the risk of diabetes mellitus and metabolic syndrome is increasing worldwide, reaching epidemic proportions.[1] At the same time, life expectancy continues to rise with the advancement of medical technologies, improved hygiene, and better access to treatments with focus on preventative therapies and the use of pharmacotherapy.[2] As a result, the survival of patients with diabetes mellitus is improving and health care providers are likely to be faced with elderly patients with diabetes, both type 1 diabetes (T1DM) and type 2 diabetes (T2DM), with increasing frequency. These patients represent a unique population because of multiple factors that health care providers should be cognizant of when making diagnostic and therapeutic decisions.

Vitally important to consider when managing elderly patients with diabetes are risk of hypoglycemia and evaluation of hypoglycemia unawareness, hypotension, risk of falls, cognitive impairment, confounding comorbidities, sarcopenia, and the higher

North Florida Integrative Medicine, Silverleaf Office Park, 6228 Northwest 43rd Street, Suite B, Gainesville, FL 32653, USA
E-mail address: nfimashleymudra@gmail.com

Physician Assist Clin 5 (2020) 247–258
https://doi.org/10.1016/j.cpha.2019.11.009   **physicianassistant.theclinics.com**

probability of side effects/interactions with the use of numerous prescribed medications[3]; all of these factors plus assessing macrovascular and microvascular complications when managing these patients. The aim is to avoid doing more harm than good by setting individualized treatment targets.

We discuss the current evidence regarding treating elderly patients with T2DM, and less emphasis is given to the treatment of T1DM. Specifically, we address the potential downsides and considerations in diagnostic and therapeutic approaches compared with middle-aged adults with diabetes mellitus. At the same time, we reinforce the importance of individualized and shared decision-making therapy, as well as a holistic approach, when making clinical decisions in these patients.

WHO SHOULD WE CONSIDER AS ELDERLY PATIENTS?

There is no clear definition as to what an elderly patient is. Many guidelines define elderly by chronologic age, and in general, a person is referred to as "elderly" when aged ≥65 years, such as in the most recent 2019 Endocrine Society Clinical Practice Guidelines.[3] Although other guidelines do not provide any specific age measure, NHANES defined the term "older" adults as ≥60 years when assessing the prevalence of functional disabilities in patients with diabetes.[4] Given the multiple discrepancies in age cut offs, this article defines elderly patients as ≥65 years but acknowledging that functional status plays a key role in determining the frailty of these patients, and a case-by-case assessment should be done when facing these patients.

EPIDEMIOLOGY OF THE AGING POPULATION

As the prolongation of life expectancy continues to increase, health care providers are facing an increasing number of elderly patients with T2DM; 33% of the US population ≥65 years are classified as diabetic and about 50% meet the criteria for prediabetes.[5] In the United States, each day more than 10,000 Baby Boomers (those born between 1944 and 1964) reach age 65 years.[6] According to the US Department of Health and Human Services, the number of people aged 65 years and older increased from 37.2 million in 2006 to 49.2 million (an increase of 33%) in 2016 and is projected to almost double to 98 million in 2060.[7] Interestingly, based on recent US Census Bureau's National Population Projections, by the year 2030 all Baby Boomers will be older than age 65.[8] As a result of this, it is estimated that by 2030, 1 in every 5 residents (20% of the entire population of the United States) will be ≥65 years. Moreover, the number of people ≥85 years is projected to more than double from 6.4 million in 2016 to 14.6 million in 2040, a 129% increase.[7]

One of the results of this population aging is an increase in the prevalence of metabolic conditions, such as T2DM, hypertension, and/or dyslipidemia. The prevalence of diabetes among patients over the age of 65 years old is 33%, and more impressively another 50% have been diagnosed with prediabetes in the US population.[5] In the United States, between 1995 and 2004, the prevalence of diabetes in nursing home residents was found to have increased from 16% to 23%.[9] The incidence of new cases of diabetes in the elderly population is likely to continue to grow according to a consensus report that estimates a 4.5-fold increase from 2005 to 2050.[10] As a result of this expanding growth in the older population and the corresponding increase in the older population with diabetes, clinicians have an increasingly essential role in taking care of these patients while addressing the issues of medication management and multiple comorbidities.

DIAGNOSING AND SCREENING FOR DIABETES

There is a common misunderstanding among health care providers that elderly patients, especially the frail elderly, do not require to be screened for diabetes. This may be related to the fact that these patients usually require a higher A1c target to avoid hypoglycemia. However, current guidelines are very clear in stating that screening for diabetes should continue regardless of the age of the patients.[3] They also suggest routine screening with A1c even during hospital admissions if the patient is to benefit from treatment.[3]

The screening should be done in a similar fashion as for middle-aged adults, which includes a fasting plasma glucose and/or A1c and then a 2-h oral glucose tolerance test for those found in the prediabetes category.[3]

These recommendations are suggested especially with patients who have high-risk factors:

- First-degree relatives with diabetes
- Overweight/obese body mass index (BMI)
- High-risk ethnicity/race (African American, Latino, Native American, Asian American, Pacific Islander)
- History of cardiovascular (CV) disease
- Hypertension (blood pressure >140/90 mm Hg)
- High-density lipoprotein (HDL) <35 mg/dL and/or triglycerides greater than 250 mg/dL
- Sleep apnea
- Physical inactivity

However, practitioners should be cognizant of inaccuracy of A1c levels with comorbid conditions, such as anemia, conditions affecting lifespan of red blood cells, chronic kidney disease (CKD), chronic liver disease, and/or a recent blood transfusion. It is also important in this population to consider whether screening for diabetes is appropriate, especially if the older patient has end-stage organ failure or a terminal disease, such as cancer.[3] It is also important, when facing an elderly patient with T2DM, not to forget to have a holistic approach to these patients, as metabolic conditions usually coexist with each other. Therefore, in **Table 1**, we have summarized the most accepted screening strategies to perform in these elderly patients during a *Medicare Annual Wellness* visit and as part of standard diabetes care.[11]

ASSESSING GLYCEMIA/SETTING GLYCEMIC TARGETS AND GOALS

Over the years, trials have looked at the effects of glycemic control on CV events in middle-aged and elderly patients with T2DM. These studies suggest assessing the overall risks and benefits when determining targets, considering both life expectancy as well as the patient's chronologic age. The heterogeneity of elderly patients ranges from high functional status persons living independently with few to no complications and comorbidities to those requiring full-time assistance in a nursing home. Therefore, addressing their comorbid conditions, functional status, and life expectancy is of the upmost importance when establishing glycemic targets.

The American Diabetes Association (ADA), American Geriatrics Association, the International Diabetes Federation and the European Diabetes Working Group have all set glycemic target goals with consideration of life expectancy, general health status, risks of hypoglycemia and compliance with treatment regimens.[12] Using shared medical decisions with the practitioner and the patient, an individualized target is established; consideration of life expectancy should be combined with glycemic A1c targets:[12]

Table 1
Assessments for the elderly patient at risk of or with type 2 diabetes

General Assessment for Annual Wellness Visit	Diabetes-Specific Health Exam
• Anthropometric measurements (weight, height, BMI) • Blood pressure, heart rate • Vision and hearing • Functional status (instrumental/activity of daily living) • Screening for depression (6CIT) • Cognition assessment • Fall risk/frailty/physical performance • Tobacco/alcohol use • Medication review • Cancer screening • Comorbid conditions	• Diabetes self-management training • Medical nutrition therapy: up to 10 h first y, then 2 h/y • Neuropathy: foot exam, monofilament • Nephropathy: urine albumin:creatinine ratio, serum creatinine/eGFR • Retinopathy—eye exam with dilation by ophthalmology

Abbreviations: 6CIT, 6-item cognitive screening test; BMI, body mass index; eGFR, estimated glomerular filtration rate.

Data from LeRoith D, Biessels GJ, Braithwaite SS, et al. Treatment of Diabetes in Older Adults: An Endocrine Society Clinical Practice Guideline. *J Clin Endocrinol Metab.* 2019 May 1;104(5):1520-1574.

- Life expectancy greater than 10 years—A1c target less than 7.5%
- Life expectancy less than 10 years with medical comorbidities—A1c target less than 8%, fasting and preprandial between 160 and 170 mg/dL
- Life expectancy less than 5 years with advanced microvascular complications and/or major comorbid conditions unlikely to benefit from intensive glycemic control—A1c target 8% to 9%

Other frameworks and categories used to assess the overall health in elderly patients have been suggested. Blaum assesses the individual's chronic health conditions (<3 vs >3+), cognitive and/or visual impairment (none, mild, moderate to severe) and need for assistance with activities of daily living (ADLs) (none vs 2+) to classify functional status.[13] Blaum defined 3 health status groups based on his criteria and then developed a tool to determine the probability of benefit of treatment based on life expectancy.[14] The ADA consensus report agreed with the categories based on Blaum's conceptual framework for overall health: group 1, good health; group 2, complex/intermediate health; and group 3, very complex/poor health.[15] The ADA criteria is helpful when determining if aggressive therapy may be successful or harmful (without the benefit of reducing complications) for the older patient. **Table 2** summarizes the recommendations given by the Endocrine Society in their most recent 2019 guidelines; categorizing A1c and blood glucose targets based on the above 3 categories.[3]

However, understanding the limitations of A1c measurements is important when dealing with elderly patients with T2DM. The measurement of A1c for overall glycemic status does not determine the occurrence or frequency of hypoglycemia, nor does it show one the significance of glycemic variability. One study of 40 patients ≥69 years (70% with T2DM and 93% treated with insulin) with an A1c >8% were assessed via a blinded continuous glucose monitoring device (CGM) for 3 days. The results showed 75% experienced a hypoglycemia event less than 60 mg/dL. Furthermore, 93% of these episodes were unrecognized by symptoms or finger stick glucose monitoring.[16] Another limitation of the A1c test is that, when developing targets in older patients, their comorbid conditions may interfere with the values; diagnoses, such as CKD,

Table 2
Groupings based on Blaum categories to determine clinical targets for elderly adults

Overall Health Category		Group 1: Good Health	Group 2: Intermediate Health	Group 3: Poor Health
Patient characteristics		No comorbidities Or 1–2 non-DM chronic illnesses[a] And No ADL[c] impairments and ≤1 IADL impairment	3+ Non-DM chronic illnesses[a] And/or Any one of the below: • Mild cognitive impairment • Early dementia • ≥2 IADL impairments	Any one below: • End-stage medical condition[b] • Moderate-severe dementia • ≥2 ADL impairments • Living in long-term nursing facility
		Reasonable glucose target ranges/HbA1c by group		
		Shared decision-making with individualized goal adjusted		
Diabetes medications with increased risk of causing hypoglycemia? (IE: insulin, sulfonylurea, glinides)	No	• Fasting: 90–130 mg/dL • Bedtime: 90–150 mg/dL • A1c <7.5%	• Fasting: 90–150 mg/dL • Bedtime: 100–180 mg/dL • A1c <8%	• Fasting: 100–190 mg/dL • Bedtime: 110–200 mg/dL • A1c 8%–8.5%[d]
	Yes	• Fasting: 90–130 mg/dL • Bedtime: 90–150 mg/dL • A1c <7.5%	• Fasting: 100–150 mg/dL • Bedtime: 150–180 mg/dL • A1c <7.5%–8%	• Fasting: 100–180 mg/dL • Bedtime: 150–250 mg/dL • A1c 8%–8.5%[d]

[a] Coexisting chronic illness (eg, osteoarthritis, chronic kidney disease stage 1–3, hypertension, stroke).

[b] One or more chronic end-stage illnesses with limited treatments and reduced life expectancy (metastatic cancer, oxygen-dependent lung disease, end-stage kidney disease, advanced heart failure).

[c] Activity of daily living (ADLs) (bathing, dressing, eating, toileting, and transferring); instrumental activity of daily living (IADLs) (preparing meals, shopping, managing money, using telephone, and managing medications).

[d] HbA1c 8.5% corresponds to average glucose level about 200 mg/dL and higher targets may result in dehydration, glycosuria, hyperglycemia crisis, and poor wound healing.

Data from LeRoith D, Biessels GJ, Braithwaite SS, et al. Treatment of Diabetes in Older Adults: An Endocrine Society Clinical Practice Guideline. *J Clin Endocrinol Metab.* 2019 May 1;104(5):1520-1574

valvular heart disease, or gastrointestinal bleeding, may alter the red blood cell turnover.

To better assess the incidence of hypoglycemia events and potentially avoid the deleterious ramifications of hypoglycemia, the use of CGMs have become a useful tool for those high-risk older patients, especially when using insulin for treatment.[3] Intermittent use of CGMs with individuals with T2DM showed a benefit for guiding treatment adjustments in antihyperglycemic drugs (excluding prandial insulin use in this study) and helped to achieve lower glycemic targets without increasing the propensity of hypoglycemia.[17] As part of the 6-month-long *Multiple Daily Injections and Continuous Glucose Monitoring in Diabetes* trial, 116 individuals older than 60 years with T1DM and T2DM who currently used multiple daily injections of insulin were randomized to using personal CGMs versus self-monitoring blood glucose.[18] The CGM group showed less glycemic variability and a greater reduction in A1c levels.[18]

TREATMENT OF HYPERGLYCEMIA
Lifestyle Interventions

Lifestyle modifications are the first line treatment of hyperglycemia for patients ≥65 years with diabetes.[3] For the prediabetic older population, metformin is not Food and Drug Administration- approved for the prevention of development of frank diabetes. Assessing the nutritional status with validated tools, such as the Mini Nutritional Assessment or Short Nutritional Assessment Questionnaire, may also assess for malnutrition.[3] Restrictive diets are not recommended in older patients with diabetes, or in those who are frail or have a risk of malnutrition or sarcopenia. Instead limiting simple sugars, and encouraging food choices to those foods rich in protein, and those that are nutrient dense and energy producing, to promote overall health are suggested.[3]

Drug Therapy for Hyperglycemia

Glycemic management should be individualized for the older patient with diabetes when choosing diabetic drug classes, especially in the setting of CKD and CV disease. The newest guidelines recommend lifestyle management followed by metformin as the first oral medication for those patients without significantly impaired kidney function (estimated glomerular filtration rate <30 mL/min/1.73 m^2) or gastrointestinal intolerance.[3] Metformin monotherapy has not been associated with an increased 5-year mortality compared with matched controls, whereas other therapy combinations (sulfonylurea [SU] + insulin had the highest mortality risk) and does not cause hypoglycemia or weight gain.[19,20] Clinical concerns of metformin therapy include the risk of lactic acidosis (usually occurring with incidents of acute kidney injury (AKI) caused by radiocontrast dye, nephrotoxic drugs, hypotension, heart failure, and so forth), and the association with vitamin B12 deficiency.[21]

Oral agents that can cause hypoglycemia and weight gain include SUs and glinides (repaglinide and nateglinide). It is recommended to avoid glyburide in older individuals. The risks of hypoglycemia with glyburide is higher when compared with the other 2 agents in the SU class: glimepiride and glipizide.[22]

Thiazolidinediones (TZDs), which include pioglitazone and rosiglitazone, have been shown to increase risks of fractures and bone loss in women and are therefore concerning for older women with osteoporosis.[23] TZDs can also cause fluid retention and thereby are contraindicated in patients with class III and IV heart failure.[24,25]

The α-glucosidase inhibitors have been shown to have only modest efficacy of glycemic control while having a relatively high rate of nonadherence due to gastrointestinal intolerance (flatulence and diarrhea).[26]

Dipeptidyl peptidase-4 inhibitors are considered weight neutral and generally well tolerated with lower risk of hypoglycemia compared with other drug classes. Previous concerns of increased risk of pancreatitis with the use of these incretin-based drugs seem not to be associated as once thought.[27]

A newer drug class, sodium-glucose cotransporter 2 (SGLT2i) inhibitors, have been shown to effectively lower A1c and increase weight loss without the risk of causing hypoglycemia. Recent studies with empagliflozin and canagliflozin have shown CV benefit by reducing major adverse cardiovascular events (MACE), heart failure, and the progression of CKD.[28,29] Given the concerns of dehydration more likely in the elderly patient population because of increased urine output, the dosing of canagliflozin should be lower.[30] One must monitor for signs of the rare occurrence of euglycemia diabetic ketoacidosis and a questionable increased incidence of lower extremity amputations (LEAs).[29,31] However, these medications are the treatment of choice in the CKD population according to the most recent ADA update on diabetic nephropathy recommendations from June 2019 based on the CREDENCE (Canagliflozin and Renal Events in Diabetes with Established Nephropathy Clinical Evaluation) trial showing a 34% lower composite risk of end-stage renal disease, doubling of serum creatinine levels, and death from renal causes, making them useful in older patients with diabetes.[32]

Glucagon-like peptide 1 (GLP-1) receptor agonists have been shown to suppress appetite, decrease glucagon secretion, delay gastric emptying, increase insulin levels, all without causing hypoglycemia events.[33] Nausea is the major side effect of this class of medication.[33] Two of the GLP-1 receptors (liraglutide and semaglutide) have been shown to improve CV outcomes.[34]

Insulin therapy is usually initiated when oral medications are not effectively controlling glycemic levels. To improve fasting glucose levels a single, long-acting basal insulin analog can be added.[35,36] If fasting blood glucose levels are in target but A1c still remains elevated, adding a prandial rapid-acting insulin before the largest meal is implemented.[35,36] The use of premixed insulins given twice daily have been developed as simpler regimens; however, they can increase risk of hypoglycemia.[36,37]

In the most recent iteration of the ADA guidelines, the use of GLP-1 agonists and SGLT2i can be prescribed earlier in the diagnosis of diabetes given their CV benefits, following metformin.[38] Practitioners, when managing elderly patients with T2DM, should keep treatment regimens simple to improve adherence, consider the risks and benefits of each of the drug classes, and consider the current cognitive status, functional status, and comorbidities while minimizing hypoglycemia.

TREATMENT OF DIABETES COMPLICATIONS IN THE ELDERLY

Older patients with T2DM (65–85 years) should be treated to a blood pressure target of 140/90 mm Hg.[3] This is to decrease risks of CV disease, stroke, and worsening CKD.[3] Those patients with prior history of stroke or worsening CKD can be considered for lower blood pressure targets (<130/80 mm Hg), with close monitoring for hypotension, syncope, electrolyte abnormalities, and/or AKI.[3] Patients with poor health (see **Table 2**) can have loosened blood pressure goals; 145 to 160/90 mm Hg. In older patients with diabetes and hypertension, the most recent guidelines recommend angiotensin-converting enzyme inhibitor (ACEi) or angiotensin receptor blockers (ARBs) as first line treatment. This is not different than recommendations for the younger aged diabetes population as these medications decrease both CKD progression and CV mortality.[3] ACEi specifically have been shown to reduce the risk of all-cause CV disease mortality, MACE, heart failure, and to reduce progression of retinopathy. ARBs significantly reduce risk of heart failure and are renoprotective.[38] For a second antihypertension treatment option, amlodipine, a calcium channel blocker, has been shown to benefit CV outcomes compared with other agents.[39]

Managing hyperlipidemia in the elderly patient population via annual lipid screening and statin therapy are recommended; however, the Endocrine Society Clinical Guidelines do not have any specific low-density lipoprotein (LDL) targets.[3] Some studies have shown adding ezetimibe to statin therapy helps lower LDL levels.[40] For the statin-intolerant patient, ezetimibe or PCSK9 inhibitors have been shown to be effective in lowering LDL levels to target (cardiology defined outcomes) and reduce CV disease outcomes.[41] The recommended first-line treatment for severe fasting hypertriglyceridemia (>500 mg/dL) in patients with diabetes is fish oil and/or fenofibrate to avoid the increased risk of pancreatitis.[3]

The treatment for primary prevention of CV events in older patients with diabetes can be challenging given the variety of functional status, multiple comorbidities, and life expectancy in this group. The use of aspirin for primary prevention continues to be an individualized choice between the practitioner and patient given both significant reductions in vascular events but also significant increased risk of major bleeding occurrences.[42]

Diabetic neuropathy is correlated with increasing age, higher A1c, and longer duration of diabetes. Thus, all older patients with diabetes should be evaluated for neuropathy to decrease amputations and the potential risks of falls and development of foot ulcers.[43,44] The prevalence of peripheral neuropathy has been shown to vary from 6% to 51% among adults with diabetes depending on their age, duration of disease, glycemia control, and the type of diabetes.[45] The risk of developing a foot ulcer has been estimated to be at 25% and LEAs are associated with diabetic peripheral neuropathy.[45] LEAs reduce quality of life, increase the risk of mortality, and increase medical costs.[46] Diabetes is the leading cause of nontraumatic LEAs according to the Centers for Disease Control and Prevention in the United States, accounting for 45% to 70% of all nontraumatic amputations. Approximately half of the diabetes-related LEAs occur among persons aged ≥65 years.[47] The risk of amputation for patients with diabetes increases due to:

- Peripheral neuropathy
- Peripheral vascular disease
- Infection/poor wound healing[47]

Because of increasing longevity, amputations in the elderly have increased, and by 2050 it is projected that the number of patients living with limb loss will more than double to 3.6 million compared with 2005.[48] Referrals for preventative foot/limb care to podiatry, fracture, and/or vein evaluations to orthopedic/vascular surgeons and referral to physical therapy for gait stability are essential in the older patient with diabetes. Minimizing medications that can potentially promote hypoglycemia, over sedation and orthostasis are important but more so in this population given their increased risk of falls and fractures.[49]

Diabetic retinopathy is an important microvascular complication in elderly patients as it can negatively impact not only their quality of life, but their ability to drive and to live independently. Subjects in the intensive control group that were enrolled in the Action to Control Cardiovascular Risk in Diabetes trial showed a 30% reduction of progression of retinopathy; however, functional status was not assessed for overall health impact.[50] Another trial, the Fenofibrate Intervention and Event Lowering in Diabetes, showed a lower incidence in the need for laser treatment for diabetic retinopathy when fenofibrates were used by older patients with diabetes.[51]

MANAGEMENT OF DIABETES AWAY FROM HOME FOR ELDERLY

It is estimated that although more than 25% of people ≥65 years have diabetes, the incidence for those living in long-term care facilities is higher at 35%.[37,38] When determining glycemic targets for patients who are either inpatients or in nursing homes, glucose levels of fasting 100 to 140 mg/dL and 140 to 180 mg/dL postprandially without causing significant hypoglycemia are the goal.[3,52] Long-term goals can then be assessed. Proper communication with the patient, family support, and medical providers involved in patient care is of the upmost important factors in transitioning care.[53]

SUMMARY

As the prevalence of diabetes mellitus increases in the general population, as well as in the elderly population as the Baby Boomers approach the age of ≥65 years, health care providers are facing a higher demand to manage diabetes and its comorbidities and complications. The benefits of glycemic control in the elderly population should be weighed against the adverse effects of antihyperglycemic medications, overall health, comorbidities/complications, life expectancy, and functional/mental status of the patient.[15] Frequently assessing the older patient for hypoglycemia, fall risk, and cognitive impairment is essential for determining their individualized treatment goals of glycemic in a shared decision-making approach.

DISCLOSURES

Nothing to disclose.

REFERENCES

1. World Health Organization. Obesity and overweight. Available at: https://www.who.int/news-room/fact-sheets/detail/obesity-and-overweight. Accessed July 4, 2019.
2. Brown GC. Living too long: the current focus of medical research on increasing the quantity, rather than the quality, of life is damaging our health and harming the economy. EMBO Rep 2015;16(2):137–41.
3. LeRoith D, Biessels GJ, Braithwaite SS, et al. Treatment of diabetes in older adults: an Endocrine Society Clinical Practice guideline. J Clin Endocrinol Metab 2019;104(5):1520–74.
4. Kalyani RR, Saudek CD, Brancati FL, et al. Association of diabetes, comorbidities, and A1C with functional disability in older adults: results from the National Health and Nutrition Examination Survey (NHANES), 1999-2006. Diabetes Care 2010;33:1055–60.
5. Menke A, Casagrande S, Geiss L, et al. Prevalence of and trends in diabetes among adults in the United States, 1988-2012. JAMA 2015;314(10):1021–9.
6. Song Z, Ferris TG. Baby Boomers and beds: a demographic challenge for the ages. J Gen Intern Med 2018;33(3):367–9.
7. US Department of Health and Human Services. Administration on aging. 2017 Profile of older Americans. Available at: https://acl.gov/sites/default/files/Aging

%20and%20Disability%20in%20America/2017OlderAmericansProfile.pdf.   Accessed July 4, 2019.

8. US Census Bureau: older people projected to outnumber children for the first time in US history. 2018. Available at: https://www.census.gov/newsroom/press-releases/2018/cb18-41-population-projections.html. Accessed July 5, 2019.

9. Zhang X, Decker FH, Luo H, et al. Trends in the prevalence and comorbidities of diabetes mellitus in nursing home residents in the United States: 1995–2004. J Am Geriatr Soc 2010;58(4):724–30.

10. Kirkman MS, Briscoe VJ, Clark N, et al. Diabetes in older adults: a consensus report. Consensus Development Conference on Diabetes and Older Adults. J Am Geriatr Soc 2012;60(12):2342–56.

11. Medicare Interactive. Annual wellness visit. Available at: www.medicareinteractive. org/get-answers/medicare-covered-services/preventive-services/annual-wellness-visit. Accessed July 2, 2019.

12. Yakaryılmaz FD, Öztürk ZA. Treatment of type 2 diabetes mellitus in the elderly. World J Diabetes 2017;8(6):278–85.

13. Blaum C, Cigolle CT, Boyd C, et al. Clinical complexity in middle-aged and older adults with diabetes: the Health and Retirement Study. Med Care 2010;48(4): 327–34.

14. Cigolle CT, Kabeto MU, Lee PG, et al. Clinical complexity and mortality in middle-aged and older adults with diabetes. J Gerontol A Biol Sci Med Sci 2012;67(12): 1313–20.

15. Kirkman MS, Briscoe VJ, Clark N, et al. Diabetes in older adults. Diabetes Care 2012;35(12):2650–64.

16. Munshi MN, Segal AR, Suhl E, et al. Frequent hypoglycemia among elderly patients with poor glycemic control. Arch Intern Med 2011;171(4):362–4.

17. Vigersky RA, Fonda SJ, Chellappa M, et al. Short- and long-term effects of real-time continuous glucose monitoring in patients with type 2 diabetes. Diabetes Care 2012;35(1):32–8.

18. Ruedy KJ, Parkin CG, Riddlesworth TD, et al. DIAMOND Study Group. Continuous glucose monitoring in older adults with type 1 and type 2 diabetes using multiple daily injections of insulin: results from the DIAMOND trial. J Diabetes Sci Technol 2017;11(6):1138–46.

19. Claesen M, Gillard P, De Smet F, et al. Mortality in individuals treated with glucose-lowering agents: a large, controlled cohort study. J Clin Endocrinol Metab 2016;101(2):461–9.

20. Holman RR, Paul SK, Bethel MA, et al. 10-Year follow-up of intensive glucose control in type 2 diabetes. N Engl J Med 2008;359(15):1577–89.

21. Chapman LE, Darling AL, Brown JE. Association between metformin and vitamin B12 deficiency in patients with type 2 diabetes: a systematic review and meta-analysis. Diabetes Metab 2016;42(5):316–27.

22. Shorr RI, Ray WA, Daugherty JR, et al. Individual sulfonylureas and serious hypoglycemia in older people. J Am Geriatr Soc 1996;44(7):751–5.

23. Zhu ZN, Jiang YF, Ding T. Risk of fracture with thiazolidinediones: an updated meta-analysis of randomized clinical trials. Bone 2014;68:115–23.

24. Nesto RW, Bell D, Bonow RO, et al. Thiazolidinedione use, fluid retention, and congestive heart failure: a consensus statement from the American Heart Association and American Diabetes Association. Diabetes Care 2004;27(1):256–63.

25. Gilbert RE, Krum H. Heart failure in diabetes: effects of anti-hyperglycaemic drug therapy. Lancet 2015;385(9982):2107–17.

26. Josse RG, Chiasson JL, Ryan EA, et al. Acarbose in the treatment of elderly patients with type 2 diabetes. Diabetes Res Clin Pract 2003;59(1):37–42.
27. Thomsen RW, Pedersen L, Møller N, et al. Incretin-based therapy and risk of acute pancreatitis: a nationwide population-based case-control study. Diabetes Care 2015;38(6):1089–98.
28. Wanner C, Inzucchi SE, Lachin JM, et al. EMPA-REG OUTCOME Investigators. Empagliflozin and progression of kidney disease in type 2 diabetes. N Engl J Med 2016;375(4):323–34.
29. Neal B, Perkovic V, Mahaffey KW, et al, CANVAS Program Collaborative Group. Canagliflozin and cardiovascular and renal events in type 2 diabetes. N Engl J Med 2017;377(7):644–57.
30. Gilbert RE, Weir MR, Fioretto P, et al. Impact of age and estimated glomerular filtration rate on the glycemic efficacy and safety of canagliflozin: a pooled analysis of clinical studies. Can J Diabetes 2016;40(3):247–57.
31. Erondu N, Desai M, Ways K, et al. Diabetic ketoacidosis and related events in the canagliflozin type 2 diabetes clinical program. Diabetes Care 2015;38(9):1680–6.
32. Perkovic V, Jardine MJ, Neal B, et al. Canagliflozin and renal outcomes in type 2 diabetes and nephropathy. N Engl J Med 2019;380(24):2295–306.
33. Zaccardi F, Htike ZZ, Webb DR, et al. Benefits and harms of once-weekly glucagon-like peptide-1 receptor agonist treatments: a systematic review and network meta-analysis. Ann Intern Med 2016;164(2):102–13.
34. Marso SP, Daniels GH, Brown-Frandsen K, et al, LEADER Steering Committee; LEADER Trial Investigators. Liraglutide and cardiovascular outcomes in type 2 diabetes. N Engl J Med 2016;375(4):311–22.
35. Inzucchi SE, Bergenstal RM, Buse JB, et al. Management of hyperglycemia in type 2 diabetes, 2015: a patient-centered approach: update to a position statement of the American Diabetes Association and the European Association for the Study of Diabetes. Diabetes Care 2015;38(1):140–9.
36. Wallia A, Molitch ME. Insulin therapy for type 2 diabetes mellitus. JAMA 2014; 311(22):2315–25.
37. Holman RR, Farmer AJ, Davies MJ, et al, 4-T Study Group. Three-year efficacy of complex insulin regimens in type 2 diabetes. N Engl J Med 2009;361(18): 1736–47.
38. Brenner BM, Cooper ME, DeZeeuw D, et al. Effects of losartan on renal and cardiovascular outcomes in patients with type 2 diabetes and nephropathy. N Engl J Med 2001;345:861–9.
39. Jamerson K, Weber MA, Bakris GL, et al. ACCOMPLISH Trial Investigators. Benazepril plus amlodipine or hydrochlorothiazide for hypertension in high-risk patients. N Engl J Med 2008;359(23):2417–28.
40. Pokharel Y, Chinnakondepalli K, Vilain K, et al. Impact of ezetimibe on the rate of cardiovascular-related hospitalizations and associated costs among patients with a recent acute coronary syndrome: results from the IMPROVE-IT Trial (Improved Reduction of Outcomes: Vytorin Efficacy International Trial). Circ Cardiovasc Qual Outcomes 2017;10(5):e003201.
41. Robinson JG, Farnier M, Krempf M, et al, ODYSSEY LONG TERM Investigators. Efficacy and safety of alirocumab in reducing lipids and cardiovascular events. N Engl J Med 2015;372(16):1489–99.
42. Bowman L, Mafham M, Wallendszus K, et al, ASCEND Study Collaborative Group. Effects of aspirin for primary prevention in persons with diabetes mellitus. N Engl J Med 2018;379(16):1529–39.

43. Popescu S, Timar B, Baderca F, et al. Age as an independent factor for the development of neuropathy in diabetic patients. Clin Interv Aging 2016;11:313–8.
44. Hicks CW, Selvin E. Epidemiology of peripheral neuropathy and lower extremity disease in diabetes. Curr Diab Rep 2019;19(10):86.
45. Narres M, Kvitkina T, Claessen H, et al. Incidence of lower extremity amputations in the diabetic compared with the non-diabetic population: a systemic review. PLoS One 2017;12(8):e0182081.
46. Centers for Disease Control and Prevention. Diabetes-related amputations of lower extremities in the Medicare population. Morb Mortal Wkly Rep 2001; 50(43):954–8. Available at: https://now.aapmr.org/lower-limb-amputations-epidemiology-and-assessment/#references.
47. Ziegler-Graham K, MacKenzie E, Ephraim PL, et al. Estimating the prevalence of limb loss in the United States: 2005 to 2050. Arch Phys Med Rehabil 2008;89: 422–9.
48. Adler AI, Boyko E, Ahroni JH, et al. Risk factors for diabetic peripheral sensory neuropathy. Results of the Seattle Prospective Diabetic Foot Study. Diabetes Care 1997;20(7):1162–7.
49. Mayne D, Stout NR, Aspray TJ. Diabetes, falls and fractures. Age Ageing 2010; 39(5):522–5.
50. Chew EY, Davis MD, Danis RP, et al. The effects of medical management on the progression of diabetic retinopathy in persons with type 2 diabetes: the Action to Control Cardiovascular Risk in Diabetes (ACCORD) Eye Study. Ophthalmology 2014;121(12):2443–51.
51. Keech AC, Mitchell P, Summanen PA, et al. FIELD Study Investigators. Effect of fenofibrate on the need for laser treatment for diabetic retinopathy (FIELD study): a randomised controlled trial. Lancet 2007;370(9600):1687–97.
52. Munshi MN, Florez H, Huang ES, et al. Management of diabetes in long-term care and skilled nursing facilities: a position statement of the American Diabetes Association. Diabetes Care 2016;39(2):308–18.
53. Newton CA, Adeel S, Sadeghi-Yarandi S, et al. Prevalence, quality of care, and complications in long term care residents with diabetes: a multicenter observational study. J Am Med Dir Assoc 2013;14(11):842–6.

The Rising Cost of Sugar
Insulin in the 21st Century

Kristen A. Scheckel, PA-C

KEYWORDS

- Cost of diabetes • Insulin costs • Insulin distribution • Global diabetes costs
- Strategies to lower diabetes costs

KEY POINTS

- Since insulin was developed the cost has progressively increased, resulting in many persons with diabetes having difficulty accessing this critical medication.
- Issues from the lack of access to insulin is a global problem and results in higher rates of diabetic complications: increased rates of diabetic ketoacidosis, longer hospital stays, and increased mortality.
- Medication and health care access are controlled by 3 domains: government, private sector, and the plural domain comprising communities and nonprofit organizations advocating for social welfare.
- There need to be significant changes within the insulin payment and distribution web, with better transparency and lower prices for patients with diabetes.

INTRODUCTION

The cost associated with diabetes care and medication treatment is a global and domestic problem. In 2015, the global cost of diabetes care was US$1.3 trillion. By 2030, the global cost is estimated to surpass $2.1 trillion.[1]

In the United States, 1 in 4 health care dollars is spent on diabetes care.[2,3] Costs of United States medical care for diabetes were estimated at $116 billion in 2007, $176 billion in 2012, and $237 billion in 2017. Other yearly indirect costs in the United States are estimated at $3.3 billion in lost revenue from work absences, $26.9 billion from reduced work productivity, and $37.5 billion from inability to work.[2,3]

EVOLUTION OF INSULIN'S RISING COST

In 1922, the insulin patent from the University of Toronto was sold for $1 with the hope that affordable insulin would cure diabetes.[4] For the first 60 years after insulin was discovered, all insulins were derived from beef or pork. Today, beef and pork insulins are no longer available in the United States.[5]

Creekside Endocrine Associates, 4101 East Louisiana Avenue, Suite 200, Denver, CO 80246, USA
E-mail address: creeksideendocrine@yahoo.com

Physician Assist Clin 5 (2020) 259–272
https://doi.org/10.1016/j.cpha.2019.11.010
2405-7991/20/© 2019 Elsevier Inc. All rights reserved.

In 1983, the first recombinant human insulin was approved by the US Food and Drug Administration (FDA) and cost $14 per vial.[4,5] Then, in 1996, the first rapid-acting insulin analog was approved and cost $24 per vial (prices not adjusted for inflation).[4] Over the next 20 years, multiple rapid-acting, long-acting, and ultralong-acting insulin analogs were approved.[5]

In 2001, human NPH insulin cost $25 per vial and glargine $44 per vial.[5] By the end of 2016, human NPH and regular insulins cost $26 per vial as the Walmart Reli-On brand, while glargine cost $298 per vial (**Fig. 1**).[5]

GLOBAL ISSUES OF INSULIN INACCESSIBILITY

To access medication, it must be available and affordable. Globally, the main cause of mortality for a patient with type 1 diabetes mellitus (T1DM) is lack of access to insulin.[6] In sub-Saharan Africa, the life expectancy of a child with T1DM is ≤1 year because of limited access to insulin.[7]

In low-income and middle-income countries, people have difficulty both affording insulin and finding it within their health care system.[6] In the Prospective Urban Rural Epidemiology (PURE) study, 156,625 participants aged 35 to 70 were recruited from 22 countries and insulin availability and cost data were collected. The study estimated that 2.8% of households in high-income countries and 63.0% of households in low-income countries could not afford insulin[8] and also found significant discrepancies in insulin availability between countries, which is summarized in **Table 1**.[8]

ISSUES REGARDING ACCESS TO INSULIN IN THE UNITED STATES

In the United States the cost of insulin is a major reason for patients to discontinue it, thus contributing to the incidence of diabetic ketoacidosis, especially in low-income populations.[7] A study conducted by Yale Diabetes Center in 2017 found that more than one-fourth of patients surveyed reported insulin underuse related to cost, which led to poor glycemic control; more than one-third of the patients did not discuss this issue with their clinician.[9]

FUTURE INSULIN NEEDS

Estimates suggest that globally the number of patients with diabetes (20–79 years old) will increase by greater than 50% by 2040.[1] Global insulin use is estimated to increase by more than 20% by 2030.[10] The production is not expected to keep up with the demand (**Fig. 2**).

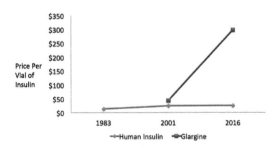

Fig. 1. Price change for human insulin versus glargine. The price of human insulin has remained relatively stable since 1983. On the other hand, the price of glargine has risen significantly since 2001. (*Data from* McEwen LN, Casagrande SS, Kuo S, Herman WH. Why are diabetes medications so expensive and what can be done to control their cost? *Curr Diab Rep.* 2017;17(9):71.)

Table 1 Differences in insulin availability between countries	
Percentage of Pharmacies Carrying Insulin (%)	Country Type
93.8	High-income countries (Canada, Saudi Arabia, Sweden, and United Arab Emirates)
76.1	India
40.2	Upper middle-income countries (Argentina, Brazil, Chile, Malaysia, Poland, South Africa, Turkey, and Russia)
29.3	Lower middle-income countries (China, Colombia, Iran, Palestinian territory, and Philippines)
10.3	Lower-income countries (Bangladesh, India, Pakistan, Tanzania, and Zimbabwe)

These data were obtained from the PURE study from 2001 to 2017 and show discrepancies in the percentage of pharmacies with insulin available.

Data from Chow CK, Ramasundarahettige C, Hu W, et al. Availability and affordability of essential medicines for diabetes across high-income, middle-income, and low-income countries: a prospective epidemiologic study. *Lancet Diabetes Endocrinol.* 2018;6(10):798-808.

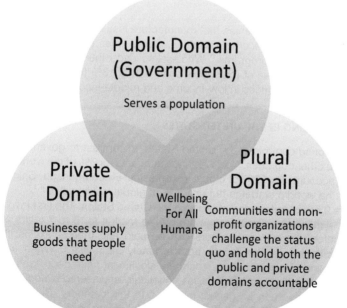

Fig. 2. Three domains controlling access to health care. The public, private, and plural domains each contribute to society's ability to access health care services and medications. (*Data from* Beran D, Hirsch IB, Yudkin JS. Why are we failing to address the issue of access to insulin? A national and global perspective. *Diabetes Care.* 2018;41(6):1125-1131.)

ECONOMIC FACTORS AFFECTING THE COST OF INSULIN
The Public Domain (Government)

The role of government is to protect the population it serves. The World Health Organization estimates that countries need to spend a minimum of US$44 per person per year to provide basic health-related services. In 2011, there were 26 low-income to middle-income countries that spent less than that amount because of limited resources. Total health spending in the United States is 214 times that minimum amount, but compared with other high-income countries the United States has worse health outcomes because of inequalities in distribution.[6]

The Private Domain ("Big Pharma")

Currently only 3 multinational pharmaceutical companies (Sanofi, Novo Nordisk, and Eli Lilly) control 99% of the insulin market.[8]

The Plural Domain (Communities and Nonprofit Organizations Advocating for Social Well-Being)

The role of the plural sector is challenge the status quo, address imbalances, and hold governments and private domains accountable. Examples of national and international associations constituting the plural sector are the International Diabetes Federation, American Diabetes Association (ADA), and Juvenile Diabetes Research Foundation.[6] Social media provide an opportunity for patients with diabetes to have their voices heard. There have been attempts in the United States to bring class action lawsuits against insulin manufacturers to decrease prices and increase accessibility.[6]

GLOBAL PRICING OF INSULIN

The 3 pharmaceutical companies that manufacture insulin have differential pricing in low-income and middle-income countries. Some offer donation programs along with patient assistance programs.[6] Wholesalers and other intermediaries increase the price at different levels of the supply chain with a 13% to 59% markup between wholesaler and patient prices in low-income and middle-income countries.[6]

MEDICATION PRICING IN THE UNITED STATES

There are no price controls in the United States, in contrast to government-run systems in some other countries. North America accounts for 7% of the world's diabetes; however, it accounts for 52% of global insulin sales. By comparison, China accounts for 25% of the world's diabetes but only 4% of global insulin sales.[4,11]

There are 2 broad categories of drugs in the United States. The first involves drugs chemically synthesized. These drugs are on the market for 5 to 7 years after being launched before generic competitors can be sold and market exclusivity can be extended, with the median length approximately 12.5 years. When medications move from brand to generic status, there are significant price decreases (**Table 2**).[5]

The second category of drugs involves genetically engineered biologic drugs made from living systems such as genes; insulin is in this category. Biologic drugs are granted market exclusivity for 12 years, and only follow-on or biosimilar insulin formulations can be approved as competitors.[5]

In 2016, the first follow-on version of the long-acting insulin analog glargine (Basaglar) was approved by the FDA after being postponed for 30 months because of a lawsuit claiming patent infringement.[5,12] Bagaslar came to market in 2017 with a

Table 2	
Effect of generic manufacturer competition on medication pricing	
Number of Generic Manufacturers	**Percent Decrease for Generic Medication**
2	55% of the brand-name price
5	33% of the brand-name price
15	13% of the brand-name price

Number of generic manufactures refers to those who are producing the same medication.
Data from McEwen LN, Casagrande SS, Kuo S, Herman WH. Why are diabetes medications so expensive and what can be done to control their cost? *Curr Diab Rep.* 2017;17(9):71.

15% lower cost than glargine (Lantus).[12] In 2017, the FDA approved a follow-on version of the short-acting Humalog insulin analog lispro (Admelog).[12]

Follow-on biologic insulin is currently approved via the FDAs 505(b) (2) pathway.[12] In 2020, all follow-on biologics will be deemed biosimilar and the 505(b) (2) pathway will disappear. All biosimilar medications will need to be approved through the FDA's 351(k) pathway. The main difference between the 2 pathways is that a biosimilar must prove it has no clinically significant difference from the reference product, whereas follow-on products may have less robust data showing similarity with the reference product.[12] For example, Admelog follow-on insulin (approved through the 505(b) (2) pathway) was not studied in children younger than 18 years old, but is approved for use in children with T1DM between the ages of 3 and 18 years old.[12]

There are multiple other follow-on insulin products currently in development for the United States market.[12] Biocon, an Indian company's biosimilar of glargine, is the only insulin to date produced by a different manufacturer and approved by a stringent authority (Japan).[6]

HEALTH INSURANCE COMPLEXITIES
Multiple Health Insurance Plans

Almost half of Americans have health insurance provided through their employer or a family member's employer (**Fig. 3**). Medicaid is a state-specific plan covering more than 68 million (20% of the population) low-income Americans that limits out-of-pocket costs for beneficiaries. Medicare is a federal health care program for older Americans (≥65 years old), those with disabilities, and those with kidney failure. Medicare covers 14% of Americans. Direct purchasers of health care (7% of the population) can use either state insurance exchanges or deal directly with an insurance company. The Veterans' Administration (VA) and the military (active duty and Tricare) cover another 2% of the population, and 9% of Americans have no health insurance.[11]

Health Insurance Deductibles

High-deductible health insurance plans (HDHP) are becoming more prevalent in the United States. The effect of HDHP on costs and outcomes was studied in 23,493 patients aged 12 to 64 years with diabetes from 2003 to 2012. After switching to HDHP, hospitalizations decreased by 11.1% in patients with diabetes, which resulted in a 3.8% reduction in total health care costs. Adverse outcomes were unchanged in the overall HDHP population with diabetes; however, there were significant differences when the data were classified by income. Members from low-income neighborhoods (8453 members) experienced 23.5% increases in high-severity emergency department visit expenditures and a 27.4% increase in high-severity hospitalization days.[13]

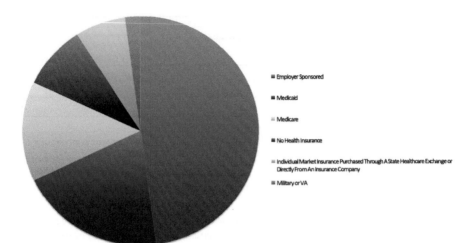

Fig. 3. Types of health insurance plans in the United States. There are multiple types of health insurance plans in the United States, listed on the right in order of greatest prevalence to lowest prevalence. (*Data from* Cefalu WT, Dawes DE, Gavlak G, et al. Insulin access and affordability working group: conclusions and recommendations. *Diabetes Care.* 2018;41(6):1299-1311.)

In a similar study involving 12,084 HDHP members with diabetes aged 12 to 64 years, the overall population with diabetes in the HDHP experienced a 49.4% increase in out-of-pocket medical expenses and an 8.0% increase in emergency room (ER) visits. The low-income subset experienced a 51.7% increase in expenses and a 21.7% increased ER visits compared with controls during the year after transitioning to the HDHP.[14]

DRUG COVERAGE AND MEDICATION PRICING IN HEALTH PLANS

Federal law requires Medicare and Medicaid to cover FDA-approved drugs, but they are prevented from negotiating lower prices. The exception is that state Medicaid programs are protected from price increases that surpass inflation, and Medicaid can receive rebates for most brand-name medications.[5]

The VA has the ability to exclude products from its formulary and is entitled to receive rebates on the medications that it chooses to include on its formulary.[5]

Pharmacy benefit managers (PBMs) are third-party administrators who negotiate with drug manufacturers and pharmacies to control drug spending and manage the prescription drug benefit plan on behalf of health insurance payers.[15] Scrutiny of PBMs has been raised because there is little regulatory oversight: they operate under private business contract law and their role in drug pricing is not transparent.[5]

PHARMACY BENEFIT MANAGERS AND DRUG COSTS

The 3 major PBMs in the United States, namely CVS Caremark, Express Scripts, and OptumRx, manage 70% of all prescription claims.[11]

Manufacturers negotiate with a PBM for discounts from the list price so as to have their medications placed on a lower and preferred cost-sharing tier. In addition, the manufacturers pay fees or rebates to the PBM after the health plan enrollees receive the medication. These retroactive rebates are in addition to the fees paid to PBMs by health insurers and other payers for their services. The retroactive rebates paid to PBMs can be as high as half the list price of insulin.[11]

Drug manufacturer rebates to PBMs increased from $39.7 billion in 2012 to $89.5 billion in 2016.[15] There is concern that the widening gap between the net and list prices of insulin are related to increasing rebates and discounts. Bloomberg News estimated that the list price of Humalog increased by 138% between 2009 and 2015 while the net price to the manufacturer increased only by 6%. Between 2001 and 2016 there was a 353% increase in the list price for a Novolog vial.[11]

When determining which drugs will be covered on a health insurance formulary, PBMs often exclude insulin made by the manufacturer that offers the lowest rebate. This results in frequent formulary changes and formulary exclusions, causing confusion for both patients and their providers (**Fig. 4**).[11]

Another controversial practice that was banned by Congress in September 2018 was a "gag clause" written by PBMs into pharmacy contracts. These clauses prohibited pharmacists from disclosing to patients that a drug may be less expensive without using insurance, thus allowing PBMs to profit from patients' co-pays.[16] A study by Van Nuys et al.[17] showed that co-payments were higher than the cash price for 1 in 4 drugs purchased by patients with Medicare Part D insurance in 2013.

MATERIAL NEED INSECURITIES

Material need insecurities refer to factors such as difficulty in paying for food, medications, housing, and/or utilities.[18]

Food insecurity can result in trade-offs between nutrition and medical care along with increased stress.[19] Up to one-fourth of United States adults with diabetes may have difficulty obtaining foods appropriate for a diabetic diet.[20] In a study of more than 41 million Americans, food insecurity for this population cost the health care system an additional $77.5 billion.[21]

Two government programs in the United States that aim to address food insecurity are the Supplemental Nutrition Assistance Program (SNAP) and the Special Supplemental Nutrition Program for Women, Infants, and Children.[22] SNAP serves approximately 1 in 7 Americans and provides food stamps to eligible participants, with eligibility criteria varying from state to state.[19]

In a retrospective cohort study of 4447 adults with income below 200% of the poverty threshold, whereby 1889 were SNAP participants and the remaining 2558 were not SNAP participants during the period 2012 to 2013, SNAP was associated with lower estimated annual health care expenses, by −$1409 on average, in fully adjusted models.[19] It has been estimated that expanding a fruits and vegetables subsidy nationwide through SNAP would reduce the incidence of T2DM by 1.7%.[23]

FOOD DESERTS

A food desert refers to an area with poor access to nutritious foods.[24] Since 2010, the federal government has incentivized full-service supermarkets to locate in low-income areas with limited access to fresh products and foods through the Healthy Food Financing Initiative.[22]

In a 2013 study in a low-income region of Pittsburgh, 571 randomly selected households that neighbored a new full-service supermarket were compared with 260 randomly selected households lacking a nearby full-service supermarket. In the neighborhood with the new supermarket, there was an 11.8% decline in food

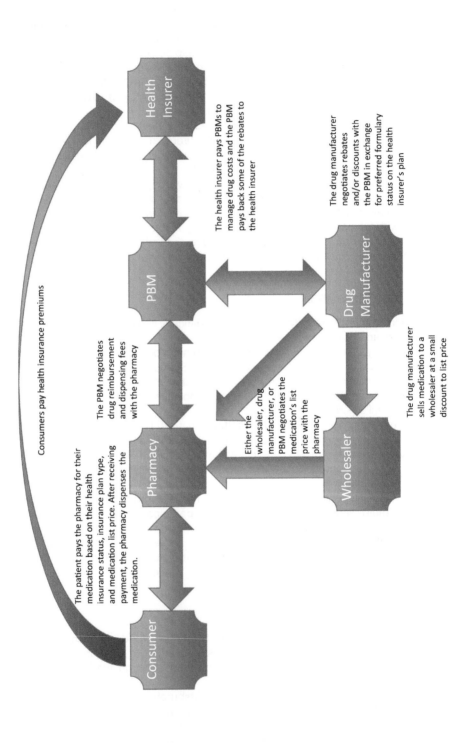

Fig. 4. Insulin payment and the distribution web, a complex system with multiple parties involved. (*Data from* Cefalu WT, Dawes DE, Gavlak G, et al.

insecurity, 9.6% fewer diagnoses of high cholesterol, and 3.6% lower prevalence of diabetes.[22]

UNSTABLE HOUSING

In a study representing more than 3 million adults with diabetes nationwide, 37% were unstably housed. Logistic regression analysis revealed that unstable housing was associated with more than 5-fold greater odds for diabetes-related ER visits or hospitalizations.[25]

HYPOGLYCEMIA COSTS

The impact of hypoglycemia on the cost of diabetes care is complex because it involves both direct costs (ie, health care resources necessary to treat hypoglycemia) and indirect costs (ie, lost productivity).[26]

For both T1DM and T2DM in the United States, hypoglycemic episodes requiring assistance from a health care provider amounted to $1161 per episode in direct costs and $160 to $176 in indirect costs. For hypoglycemic episodes requiring nonmedical assistance, the cost amounted to $66 per episode in direct costs and $242 to $579 in indirect costs. For hypoglycemic episodes managed with self-treatment, both the direct and indirect costs were $11 each.[26]

INITIATIVES TO REDUCE DIABETES EXPENDITURES
Centers for Medicare & Medicaid Services Competitive Bidding Program

The Centers for Medicare & Medicaid Services (CMS) competitive bidding program was launched in 2013 with the intention of reducing beneficiary out-of-pocket expenses. The goal is to ensure access to durable medical equipment, prosthetics, orthotics, and supplies while controlling costs. CMS has reported that competitive bidding has saved millions of dollars; however, concerns have been raised about disrupted access to diabetes supplies. This may lead to increased mortality, hospitalizations, and costs among the insulin-treated diabetes subgroup. Additional concerns are the Medicare policy limit of 3 glucometer strips per day for beneficiaries on insulin and inaccuracies in up to 45% of the glucometer systems currently covered by CMS.[27]

The National Diabetes Prevention Program

The National Diabetes Prevention Program demonstration project showed that intensive lifestyle intervention or metformin for 3 years was able to delay the onset of T2DM among high-risk adults by 58% (lifestyle) and 31% (metformin), with persistent reduction in diabetes incidence for 15 years.[28]

Currently CMS pays only $10 per patient for 30 minutes of group education and training by a nonphysician health care provider for up to 5 to 8 patients (current CPT code 98962).[28] A demonstration project from the Montefiore Health System in New York estimated that the true cost of these classes is $88.71 per patient per session. Present reimbursement from Medicare is insufficient.[28]

Medicare Shared Savings Program

In 2012, the Rio Grande Valley Accountable Care Organization (ACO) Heath Providers LLC in Donna, Texas joined CMS in the Medicare Shared Savings Program. Using a team approach with patient care coordinators, physicians, physician assistants, nurse practitioners, diabetes educators, and nutritionists, they were able to show a significant decrease in ER visits and hospital admissions. The shared savings ranged from $12 million to 21.6 million annually.[29]

Medicaid Expansion

In states that expanded Medicaid eligibility from 2014 to 2015, there were 30 additional diabetes prescriptions filled annually per 1000 population in comparison with states that did not expand Medicaid eligibility. Prescriptions filled for insulin increased by 40% after Medicaid expansion. Further expansion of Medicaid eligibility may address gaps in access to diabetes medications.[30]

OTHER INITIATIVES
Intensive Lifestyle Interventions

The Action for Health in Diabetes (Look AHEAD) trial used intensive lifestyle interventions for weight loss in patients with T2DM and reduced individual health care costs by nearly $5300 over 10 years.[31,32]

Medically Tailored Meal Delivery

Geisinger Health Systems created a "Farmacy" program that provides meals and diabetes education free of charge to patients and their families dealing with food insecurity. In an 18-month period, participants in the "Farmacy" program experienced a 2.1% decrease in their hemoglobin A1c, whereas patients on medications alone experienced only a 0.5% to 1.2% decrease in their hemoglobin A1c.[33]

Individualizing Patients' Medication

Health care providers have the option of prescribing less expensive generic insulin.[34] There are also patient assistance programs offered by manufacturers with various eligibility requirements that vary according to the individual's income, state, medication, and health insurance coverage.[4]

Cost Sharing for Insulin

It has been estimated that eliminating cost sharing for all insulins would save patients an average of $430 per patient per year in out-of-pocket costs. This would increase insurance premiums by only $2.63 to $5.23 per member per year.[35]

American Diabetes Association

In 2017, the ADA formed an insulin access and affordability task force. The ADA advocates for changes in the law to help protect persons with diabetes against rising medication costs and has identified the following steps to improve insulin access and affordability.

1. Transparency within the insulin supply chain should be improved.
2. Health care providers, pharmacies, and insurance plans should help those with diabetes understand medical and financial implications of the different insulin preparations.
3. Health care providers should prescribe the lowest-priced insulin required.
4. The insulin list price should more closely reflect the net price.
5. Rebates should be used to lower insulin cost at the point of sale.
6. There is a need for research comparing the cost-effectiveness of the different insulin preparations.
7. Efforts should be made to develop more effective insulin preparations.

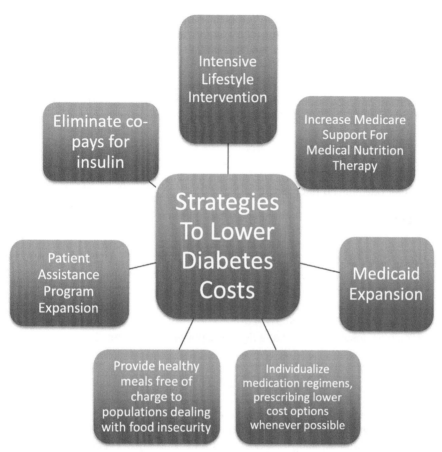

Fig. 5. Strategies to lower diabetes costs. There are multiple different ways to reduce costs associated with diabetes care and medication expense burden. (*Data from* Refs.[4,11,28,30–35])

8. The FDA should streamline the process to bring "follow-on" and "biosimilar" insulins to market (**Fig. 5**).[11]

SUMMARY

Insulin inaccessibility and the rising cost of diabetes care are troubling problems with deep consequences for society unless dramatic changes are undertaken. It is heartbreaking to realize the global magnitude of increased diabetes complications, pain, suffering, and death that result from difficulties accessing and affording insulin.

As health care providers in the United States, we should be having frank discussions with patients regarding their ability to afford their medications and working with our patients to individualize their medication regimen to help reduce their medication costs. Health care systems are increasingly accountable for the health outcomes even if the root issues are outside the scope of clinical care. This makes social determinants of health our issue. Health care systems could increase collaboration with government programs, community resources, community health workers, peer support groups, and programs providing healthy food, while making medications available at very low or no out-of-pocket cost.[18]

In high-income countries, diabetes progress is determined by novelties such as new insulin, new medications, and new technology. This does not have an impact on the majority population living with diabetes globally. We should continue to strive for new innovations but must not forget that many people with diabetes are unable to access the basic treatments such as insulin.[6]

The test of our progress is not whether we add more to the abundance of those who have much; it is whether we provide enough for those who have little
— *Franklin D. Roosevelt*[6]

DISCLOSURE

The author has nothing to disclose.

REFERENCES

1. Bommer C, Saggalova V, Hessemann E, et al. Global economic burden of diabetes in adults: projections from 2015 to 2030. Diabetes Care 2018;41(5):963–70.
2. Riddle MC, Herman WH. The cost of diabetes care—an elephant in the room. Diabetes Care 2018;41(5):929–32.
3. American Diabetes Association. Economic costs of diabetes in the U.S. in 2017. Diabetes Care 2018;41(5):917–28.
4. Hirsch IB. Insulin in America: a right or a privilege? Diabetes Spectr 2016;29(3): 130–2.
5. McEwen LN, Casagrande SS, Kuo S, et al. Why are diabetes medications so expensive and what can be done to control their cost? Curr Diab Rep 2017; 17(9):71.
6. Beran D, Hirsch IB, Yudkin JS. Why are we failing to address the issue of access to insulin? A national and global perspective. Diabetes Care 2018;41(6):1125–31.
7. Beran D, Ewen M, laing R. Constraints and challenges in access to insulin: a global perspective. Lancet Diabetes Endocrinol 2016;4(3):275–85.
8. Chow CK, Ramasundarahettige C, Hu W, et al. Availability and affordability of essential medicines for diabetes across high-income, middle-income, and low-income countries: a prospective epidemiological study. Lancet Diabetes Endocrinol 2018;6(10):798–808.
9. Herkert D, Vijayakumar P, Luo J, et al. Cost-related insulin underuse among patients with diabetes. JAMA Intern Med 2019;179(1):112–4.
10. Basu S, Yudkin JS, Kehlenbrink S, et al. Estimation of global insulin use for type 2 diabetes, 2018-30: a microsimulation analysis. Lancet Diabetes Endocrinol 2019; 7(1):25–33.
11. Cefalu WT, Dawes DE, Gavlak G, et al. Insulin access and affordability working group: conclusions and recommendations. Diabetes Care 2018;41(6):1299–311.
12. Rasmussen JT, Ipema HJ. Formulary considerations for insulins approved through the 505(b)(2) "follow-on" pathway. Ann Pharmacother 2019;53(2): 204–10.
13. Wharam JF, Zhang F, Eggleston EM, et al. Effect of high-deductible insurance on high-acuity outcomes in diabetes: a natural experiment for translation in diabetes (NEXT-D) study. Diabetes Care 2018;41(5):940–8.
14. Wharam JF, Zhang F, Eggleston EM, et al. Diabetes outpatient care and acute complications before and after high-deductible insurance enrollment: a natural

experiment for translation in diabetes (NEXT-D) study. JAMA Intern Med 2017; 177(3):358–68.

15. Pharmacy benefit managers and their role in drug spending. New York: Commonwealth Fund; 2019. Available at: https://www.commonwealthfund.org/publications/explainer/2019/apr/pharmacy-benefit-managers-and-their-role-drug-spending 10. 26099/njmh-en20. Accessed May 6, 2019.

16. Seeley E, Kesselheim AS. Pharmacy benefit managers: practices, controversies, and what lies ahead. New York: Commonwealth Fund; 2019. Available at: https://www.commonwealthfund.org/publications/issue-briefs/2019/mar/pharmacy-benefit-managers-practices-controversies-what-lies-ahead 10.26099/n60j-0886. Accessed May 6, 2019.

17. Van Nuys K, Joyce G, Ribero R, et al. Frequency and magnitude of co-payments exceeding prescription drug costs. JAMA 2018;319(10):1045–7.

18. Berkowitz SA, Meigs JB, DeWalt D, et al. Material need insecurities, control of diabetes mellitus, and use of health care resources: results of the measuring economic insecurity in diabetes study. JAMA Intern Med 2015;175(2):257–65.

19. Berkowitz SA, Seligman HK, Rigdon J, et al. Supplemental nutrition assistance program (SNAP) participation and health care expenditures among low-income adults. JAMA Intern Med 2017;177(11):1642–9.

20. Knight CK, Probst JC, Liese AD, et al. Household food insecurity and medication "scrimping" among US adults with diabetes. Prev Med 2016;83:41–5.

21. Berkowitz SA, Basu S, Meigs JB, et al. Food insecurity and health care expenditures in the United States, 2011-2013. Health Serv Res 2018;53(3):1600–20.

22. Richardson AS, Ghosh-Dastidar M, Beckman R, et al. Can the introduction of a full-service supermarket in a food desert improve residents' economic status and health? Ann Epidemiol 2017;27(12):771–6.

23. Choi SE, Seligman H, Basu S. Cost effectiveness of subsidizing fruit and vegetable purchases through the supplemental nutrition assistance program. Am J Prev Med 2017;52(5):147–55.

24. Berkowitz SA, Karter AJ, Corbie-Smith G, et al. Food insecurity, food "deserts", and glycemic control in patients with diabetes: a longitudinal analysis. Diabetes Care 2018;41(6):1188–95.

25. Berkowitz SA, Kalkhoran S, Edwards ST, et al. Unstable housing and diabetes-related emergency department visits and hospitalization: a nationally representative study of safety-net clinic patients. Diabetes Care 2018;41(5):933–9.

26. Foos V, Varol N, Curtis BH, et al. Economic impact of severe and non-severe hypoglycemia in patients with type 1 and type 2 diabetes in the United States. J Med Econ 2015;18(6):420–32.

27. Puckrein GA, Hirsch IB, Parkin CG, et al. Impact of the 2013 national rollout of CMS competitive bidding program: the disruption continues. Diabetes Care 2018;41(5):949–55.

28. Parsons AS, Raman V, Starr B, et al. Medicare underpayment for diabetes prevention program: implications for DPP suppliers. Am J Manag Care 2018; 24(10):475–8.

29. Pena JF, Penalo PJ, Estevez EF. South Texas ACO finds perfect formula: patients' diabetes outcomes were improved and millions of dollars saved. Health Exec 2017;32(2):58–60.

30. Myerson R, Lu T, Tonnu-Mihara I, et al. Medicaid eligibility expansions may address gaps in access to diabetes medications. Health Aff 2018;37(8):1200–7.

31. Benker BT, Dunn JP, Stephenson K. The rising cost of diabetes: can DiRECT tip the scales? Obesity (Silver Spring) 2018;26(12):1866–7.

32. Espeland MA, Glick HA, Bertoni A, et al. Impact of an intensive lifestyle intervention on use and cost of medical services among overweight and obese adults with type 2 diabetes: the action for health in diabetes. Diabetes Care 2014; 37(9):2548–56.

33. Feinberg AT, Hess A, Passaretti M, et al. Prescribing food as a specialty drug. NEJM Catalyst. 2018. Available at: https://catalyst.nejm.org/prescribing-fresh-food-farmacy/. Accessed June 3, 2019.

34. Zilbermint M, Schiavone L. To give or not to give: the challenge of pharmaceutical coupons. J Clin Ethics 2018;29(4):319–22.

35. Jackson EA, Berman M. Mitigating out-of-pocket costs for prescription drugs: a discussion document prepared for Eli Lilly. Seattle (WA): Milliman; 2016. Available at: http://us.milliman.com/insight/2017/Mitigating-out-of-pocket-costs-for-prescription-drugs/. Accessed March 4, 2019.

Leaving Diabetes Behind
Look How Far We've Come

Courtney Lee Bennett Wilke, MPAS, PA-C[a],*,
Brittany M. Dowdle, BA[b], Megan J. Dougan, MPAS, PA-C[c]

KEYWORDS

• Future • Diabetes • Nanomedicine • Gene therapy • Biofilter • Artificial intelligence

KEY POINTS

- Diabetes treatment has come a long way in the last hundred years, and today's innovations have improved patients' quality of life, but will the leap in the next hundred years be beyond what we can imagine?
- Diabetes treatment 100 years in the future—will technological developments eradicate diabetes for future generations?
- What might future diabetes treatments look like? From nanotechnology to advanced gene therapy, the technological advances that could be brought to bear on the treatment of diabetes hold promise for generations to come.

The year is 2120, and *diabetes* is a word that has all but vanished from our vocabulary. In this age of artificial intelligence (AI)–directed mass data analysis, worldwide universal health care, nanomedicine, and the ascendency of prevention over cure, the benefits we live with today would have seemed like far-off dreams to the average person living a hundred years ago, in 2020.

Twenty-first century "millennials" surely thought themselves well removed from the dark ages of medicine, those centuries when people with diabetes were consigned to a shortened existence marked by recurrent discomfort with virtually no medical therapy available to lessen their symptoms. These early humans suffered poor glycemic control and multiple long-term consequences of hyperglycemia, including blindness, kidney failure, amputations, gastroparesis, and coronary disease—if they managed to survive that long.

In contrast, most people living in the 2020s thought themselves in a new modern era of space-age advancements, despite the fact that millions of individuals pricked themselves daily with sharp instruments as they tried to control blood sugar levels that had already veered off goal—a barbaric practice by today's standards. And oral

[a] School of Physician Assistant Practice, College of Medicine, Florida State University, Thrasher Building 1160, Tallahassee, FL 32306-4300, USA; [b] 4971 State Highway 60, Suches, GA 30572, USA; [c] 1354 Wintergreen Lane, Fairview, PA 16415, USA
* Corresponding author.
E-mail addresses: courtney.wilke@med.fsu.edu; cbennettwilke@gmail.com

Physician Assist Clin 5 (2020) 273–276
https://doi.org/10.1016/j.cpha.2019.11.011   physicianassistant.theclinics.com

medications, although effective, were not a panacea either. Although designed to help control glucose, they were accompanied by many side effects that negatively affected patients' quality of life, causing symptoms such as nausea, hypoglycemia, and weight gain.

Eventually continuous glucose monitors and closed-loop insulin pump systems were developed, but financial constraints played a significant role in determining which patients had access to these devices, as everyday people found themselves mired in the morass of political bureaucracy and commercial interests that overshadowed that era's health care. The complexity of managing the new treatment systems was also a challenge to nonaugmented (baseline) humans, who had difficulty merging the technical know-how and their so-called smart devices, which they carried in their pockets and plugged in to the monolithic electrical grids that were standard at that time.

Although imperfect, all these small medical developments put us on the right track to the solutions that have helped us attain one of the twenty-second century's most startling medical achievements—the elimination of diabetes altogether. Consider how far we've come…

DIABETES TODAY

The year is 2120, and it is a cleaner, kinder, and safer world than the one we inherited from our twenty-first century predecessors. Not that it has been easy, or without controversy and sacrifice—some would say we've simply traded one set of world problems for another—but a look at the medical breakthroughs alone shows that most humans are healthier than at any other time in history. And the prevention (and when necessary, treatment) of diabetes is a perfect example.

Patients no longer drive to a provider's office miles from their home, lugging with them their glucometers or well-worn journals with tattered corners and nearly illegible blood sugar measurements scrawled in endless columns. Now patients with diabetes have a medical tattoo, made of electro-conductive material that monitors blood pressure, heart rate, lipid levels, and glucose levels on a virtually continuous basis. This tattoo works by interfacing with personalized nanobots that are designed to work seamlessly with each person's genetic and metabolic makeup. This allows for multilevel monitoring of the patient's biophysical profile in real time. The tattoo wirelessly communicates this data directly to an AI medical provider. The AI provider analyzes any deviance from acceptable normal ranges and works remotely with the patient's own nanobots to correct the imbalance. Regardless of the patient's nationality, language, or health care consortium affiliation, the AI has access to global anonymized metrics to help guide treatment decisions, leveraging universal health to benefit individual health.

Dietary indiscretions are no longer the bane of a diabetic patient's existence, in large part because traditional foods that have high carbohydrate content and/or elevated glycemic index have been genetically modified to consist of indigestible fibers rather than simple carbohydrates. Those food items that were unable to be modified (or were distasteful to the human palate afterward) were outlawed in most of the industrialized world in the interest of public health. In addition, as the *Slow Food* movement, which encourages nutritious, seasonal foods, gained ground in the 2040s and merged with new trends in community-supported agriculture and the widespread adoption of environmentally sustainable locally adapted farming, the dinner plate was revolutionized around the world. The highly processed, high-fat, high-sodium, low-nutrient diet made popular through twentieth-century Western culture fell out of favor, bringing about one of the most significant shifts in public health since the advent of antiseptic.

Complications from uncontrolled diabetes are now nearly unheard of, reported only anecdotally in those regions where a small and strongly independent-minded segment of the population, wary of medical technology, has assiduously avoided the universal health care available to all. There is no general awareness of diabetic amputations, neuropathy is unheard of, and the idea that a person might have a shortened life expectancy because of something called *diabetes* is ancient history.

OUR PATIENTS WITH DIABETES

Let us take a look at what remains of diabetes in the year 2120 and the progression of treatment options that are available.

Yawen is a 98-year-old woman born in 2022 and has a life expectancy of 130 years. She has early signs of hyperglycemia and diabetes and has steadfastly refused any type of "newfangled" medical intervention. But recently, Yawen was convinced by her great-grandchildren that it is time for her to embrace current medical innovation. She will receive a transcutaneous placement of a living biofilter that removes excess glucose from her bloodstream and stores it as an energy source to be used to self-regenerate, thus eliminating the need for replacement filters. The procedure is painless, effective, and avoids what she considers to be fearsome bionic nanotechnology.

Tal is a 77-year-old man born in 2043. He has what in the twenty-first century would have been called metabolic syndrome and severe insulin resistance. He too is reluctant to place himself at what he considers the mercy of new medical technologies, but he is a good candidate for a micro artificial pancreas (MAP) transplant. Created from a 3D printer, the MAP is the size of a pea and creates its own insulin from pancreatic β cells in response to ambient glucose levels. Thankfully, he does not require any immunosuppressants because the pancreas transplant generates a biofilm, making it invisible to his immune system. His family almost has him convinced that this intervention will improve his life, and with any luck, he will agree to the transplant soon.

Markus is a 54-year-old man born in 2066. He was recently found to have biomarkers suggesting that he was in the beginning stages of developing late-onset type 1 diabetes. He just received a nanobot-mediated delivery of his own pancreatic stem cells to his native pancreas. These cells were genetically altered to evade his own immune system, so that no long-term immunosuppressive therapy will be required. As his native pancreatic cells become nonfunctional, his modified pancreatic cells will continue to function at full capacity, responding to blood serum levels with insulin production.

Savannah is a 37-year-old woman born in 2083. In her prenatal screening she was found to have a biomarker for gestational insulin resistance. She was given the option to provide an extrauterine gestational environment for her fetus, but preferred to carry it fully to term in what she considered a more "natural" environment. Of the available options, she chose to have a transdermal micro biosensor implanted in her upper arm. In addition to simple monitoring of her serum glucose levels, it uses magneto-chemical technology to attract and neutralize glucose molecules, normalizing blood sugar levels. The resulting euglycemia is ideal for fetal growth while not exposing the fetus to high insulin levels or potentially disruptive nanotechnology.

Roderico is a 24-year-old man born in 2096. He was identified by genetic screening at birth as having a 92.67% chance of developing type 2 diabetes by the age of 28. He was noted to have a dysfunctional gene that would cause impaired islet cell activity. He received gene replacement therapy late last year. His dysfunctional gene was replaced with a fully functional allele, and his pancreatic insulin function remains intact.

THE LAST PATIENT WITH DIABETES

Shonya is a 6-year-old girl, brought into this world in 2114. She was genetically pro-grammed before birth based on the recommendations from the leading fertility AI, *Pro-CREATE*. Genetic analysis of her parents identified multiple genetic aberrancies that could cause health problems over the course of Shonya's lifetime, including a strong inclination toward diabetes. Rather than being condemned to a lottery of sorts, where a substantial portion of the available numbers spelled demise, genetic programming sorted through the available options to select for the genes that coded for the charac-teristics of long-term health. Although her family members were treated for diabetes over their lifespans, she will never experience diabetes herself.

WHAT THE FUTURE HOLDS

Just as the medical advances we enjoy today, in 2120—such as the virtual elimination of diabetes as a morbidity factor—seem light-years from a mere 100 years in the past, so too must we stretch our imaginations to envision life years in our future. Will space travel present medical challenges to our gravity-bound nanotechnologies and will the concomitant cosmic rays create complexities in our efforts to modify genes? What wonders will our descendants see, what worlds will they explore, and how can the work we do today ensure that they are healthy and fit for the challenges and opportu-nities that lie ahead? Whichever direction our future carries us, the ingenuity and perseverance that helped us defang diabetes will continue to embolden and empower us to overcome the obstacles ahead.

DISCLOSURE

Disclosure of any relationship with a commercial company that has a direct financial interest in subject matter or materials discussed in article or with a company making a competing product: none.

Moving?

Make sure your subscription moves with you!

To notify us of your new address, find your **Clinics Account Number** (located on your mailing label above your name), and contact customer service at:

Email: journalscustomerservice-usa@elsevier.com

800-654-2452 (subscribers in the U.S. & Canada)
314-447-8871 (subscribers outside of the U.S. & Canada)

Fax number: 314-447-8029

Elsevier Health Sciences Division
Subscription Customer Service
3251 Riverport Lane
Maryland Heights, MO 63043

*To ensure uninterrupted delivery of your subscription, please notify us at least 4 weeks in advance of move.

Printed and bound by CPI Group (UK) Ltd, Croydon, CR0 4YY

03/10/2024

01040475-0009